An Outline of Modern Psychiatry

JENNIFER HUGHES, MRCP, MRCPsych

Department of Psychiatric Medicine,
Royal South Hants Hospital, Southampton

A Wiley Medical Publication

JOHN WILEY & SONS
Chichester · New York · Brisbane · Toronto · Singapore

Library of Congress Cataloguing in Publication Data:

Hughes, Jennifer.
  An outline of modern psychiatry.

  (A Wiley medical publication)
  Includes index.
  1. Psychiatry. I. Title. II. Series.
  [DNLM: 1. Mental disorders. WM 100 H893o]

RC454.H83   616.89   81-16399
                                   AACR2

British Library Cataloguing in Publication Data:

Hughes, Jennifer
  An outline of modern psychiatry.
  1. Psychiatry
  I. Title
  616.89   RC454

ISBN 0 471 10073 0 (Cloth)
ISBN 0 471 10024 2 (Paper)

Phototypeset by Dobbie Typesetting Service, Plymouth, Devon and
printed at The Pitman Press, Bath, Avon.

Introduction

During the first years of my postgraduate training in psychiatry, I would have liked a short book which clearly summarized current knowledge of the subject, and was easy to use for reference or revision. Existing short texts contained too much elementary explanation, not enough facts, nor enough about recent research; the long ones were too detailed to be easily read as a whole, or used for rapid reference. I therefore wrote this as an adjunct to standard texts for doctors beginning postgraduate training in psychiatry, or revising for the final MRCPsych; medical students, GPs, MRCP candidates, nurses, clinical psychologists and social workers may also find it useful. The book is deliberately written in a terse, condensed style and does not attempt to discuss abstract or philosophical issues, but contains many references to original papers and longer reviews. A very detailed index is included as an aid to readers practising multiple choice questions.

Acknowledgements

I am especially grateful to Dr. Brian Barraclough, whose ideas contributed so much to this book; and to Mrs. Hazel Hills for extensive secretarial help. I should also like to thank Professor James Gibbons, Dr. David Hughes, and Dr. Jane Newson-Smith for their helpful comments on the manuscript, and Miss Betty Webb for typing early drafts.

Contents

CHAPTER 1

Classification

Classification of disease is essential as a guide to treatment and prognosis, and for the advancement of knowledge. Classification in psychiatry is based on the description of syndromes each with characteristic symptoms, signs, and course. A classification based on cause would be more satisfactory, but is not possible in the present state of knowledge. Psychiatric disorders with no known organic cause are sometimes termed 'functional'.

The ICD

The International Classification of Mental Disorders (ICD), 9th revision (World Health Organization, 1978) uses the following scheme:

ICD *No.*	*Condition*
	Organic psychotic conditions
290	Senile and presenile organic psychotic conditions
291	Alcoholic psychoses
292	Drug psychoses
293	Transient organic psychotic conditions
294	Other organic psychotic conditions (chronic)
	Other psychoses
295	Schizophrenic psychoses
296	Affective psychoses
297	Paranoid states
298	Other non-organic psychoses
299	Psychoses with origin specific to childhood
	Neurotic disorders, personality disorders, and other non-psychotic mental disorders
300	Neurotic disorders
301	Personality disorders

1

302	Sexual deviations and disorders
303	Alcohol dependence syndrome
304	Drug dependence
305	Non-dependent abuse of drugs
306	Physiological malfunction arising from mental factors
307	Special symptoms or syndromes not elsewhere classified
308	Acute reaction to stress
309	Adjustment reaction
310	Specific non-psychotic mental disorders following organic brain damage
311	Depressive disorder, not elsewhere classified
312	Disturbance of conduct not elsewhere classified
313	Disturbance of emotions specific to childhood and adolescence
314	Hyperkinetic syndrome of childhood
315	Specific delays in development
316	Psychic factors associated with disease classified elsewhere

Mental retardation
317	Mild mental retardation
318	Other specified mental retardation
319	Unspecified mental retardation

Only the 3-digit categories are listed here; the 4-digit categories provide a more detailed subdivision, but sometimes at the expense of reliability. Some conditions relevant to psychiatry are classified in other sections of the ICD, e.g. suicide and self-inflicted injury or poisoning (E950–E958).

DSM–III

A different classification, DSM–III, is used in the USA (American Psychiatric Association, 1980). DSM–III was developed from rigidly defined diagnostic criteria prepared for research use by Feighner *et al.* (1972) and expanded by Spitzer *et al.* (1975).

If the same classification was universally followed, the comparability of international statistics would be improved.

Further Reading

The place of diagnosis in psychiatry is discussed in the book by Kendell (1975).

References

American Psychiatric Association (1980). *Diagnostic and Statistical Manual of Mental Disorders*. American Psychiatric Association, Washington D.C.

Feighner, J. P., Robins, E., Guze, S. B., Woodruff, R. A., Winokur, G., and Munoz, R. (1972). Diagnostic criteria for use in psychiatric research. *Arch. Gen. Psychiatry*, **26**, 57–63.

Kendell, R. E. (1975). *The Role of Diagnosis in Psychiatry*. Blackwell Scientific Publications, Oxford.

Spitzer, R. L., Endicott, J., and Robins, E. (1975). Clinical criteria for psychiatric diagnosis and DSM-III. *Am. J. Psychiatry*, **132**, 1187–1192.

World Health Organization (1978). *Mental Disorders: Glossary and Guide to their Classification in Accordance with the Ninth Revision of the International Classification of Diseases*. WHO, Geneva.

CHAPTER 2

History-taking, Examination, and Investigation

The case history and mental state examination are the main sources of the information required to make a diagnosis in the psychiatric patient. Laboratory investigations are helpful in a minority of cases only. The case history also provides details of the patient's personality, relationships, and life circumstances, and how they have been affected by the illness; this knowledge may help to determine the method, setting, and goals of treatment chosen. The history-taking interview, which conventionally lasts one hour, may have therapeutic value in itself as it gives the patient an opportunity to express his or her problems, and it plays an important part in the establishment of the relationship between patient and psychiatrist.

History

1. *Introduction:* patient's name, age, marital status, occupation, where seen and how referred.

2. *Complaints:* in patient's own words.

3. *History of present illness:*
    (a) Duration.
    (b) Symptoms, including changes in sleep, appetite, mood, energy, and concentration.
    (c) Possible precipitating factors.
    (d) Effect of the illness on personal relationships and working efficiency.
    (e) Treatment so far.

4

4. *Family history:*

(a) Parents' and siblings' ages, occupation, health, and relationship with patient. If dead, record age and cause of death, and patient's age at the time.

(b) Family history of psychiatric illness, suicide, alcoholism.

5. *Personal history:*

(a) Childhood: a detailed account is relevant in younger patients only.

(i) complications during pregnancy or birth, serious illnesses in infancy, or delays in development (all suggesting the possibility of brain damage).

(ii) home environment: place of birth, other places of residence, emotional atmosphere and practical circumstances at home, outstanding events.

(iii) school: academic achievements, ability to mix with other children, attitude to teachers.

(iv) 'neurotic traits' e.g. nail-biting, bed-wetting (conventionally included although they do not predict adult neurosis).

(b) Work: list jobs held, with degrees of competence and satisfaction, and reasons for change. This provides information about abilities and personality, and has relevance for rehabilitation.

(c) Sexual: past and present practice, difficulties, deviations. Detailed inquiry about sexual development is not necessary unless it is relevant to the present illness.

(d) Marital: duration of marriage, spouse's age, occupation, health, and relationship with the patient. Record the same details for any previous marriages, and reasons for their termination.

(e) Children: names, ages, health, relationship with the patient.

(f) Medical history: past illnesses, present physical symptoms, treatment.

(g) Past psychiatric history: dates of previous episodes of illness, diagnosis, treatment.

6. *Premorbid personality:*

(a) Social relations: ability to make friends and relate to those in authority.

(b) Mood: cheerful or despondent, anxious or placid, tendency to mood swings, outbursts of temper, response to stress.

(c) Character: confident or diffident, independent or reliant on others, conscientious and perfectionist or otherwise.

(d) Level of energy and activity.

(e) Attitude to religion, politics, membership of groups or societies, hobbies.

(f) Alcohol and tobacco consumption, drug abuse.

(g) Criminal behaviour.

In some patients the presenting disturbance will be seen to be an exaggeration of personality problems. In others, alteration of characteristic mood and behaviour suggests an illness.

7. *Present circumstances:* type of accommodation, people in household, financial or practical problems.

Mental State Examination

1. *Appearance and general behaviour:* striking physical features (e.g. abnormal height or weight, deformities), type of dress, standard of grooming, degree of activity, abnormalities of movements or gait, whether cooperative.

2. *Talk:* the form, not the content, of talk is recorded here. Note amount, speed, whether spontaneous or only in answer to questions. Coherence: puns, rhymes, odd changes of topic or abrupt pauses. Write down a sample of talk verbatim if the form is abnormal.

3. *Mood:* patient's own description and interviewer's observations. Mood states include depression, euphoria, anxiety, perplexity, fear, suspicion. Mood may fluctuate during the interview, or be inappropriate to the circumstances or the patient's thought content.

4. *Thought content:* subjects which preoccupy the patient, and obsessive–compulsive phenomena, i.e. recurrent thoughts or actions which the patient recognizes as illogical but cannot prevent.

5. *Abnormal beliefs and experiences:* ideas of reference, delusions, passivity feelings, thought interference, depersonalization or derealization, hallucinations, illusions (see Glossary).

6. *Cognitive functioning:*

(a) Memory: long-term memory can be assessed from the history. Tests of short-term memory include the ability to repeat a name and address both immediately and after five minutes, and the digit span test (the number of digits a patient is able to repeat back to the interviewer).

(b) Orientation: in time (day, date, time of day), in place, and in person (by identification of the interviewer or ward staff).

(c) Attention and concentration: tests include ability to list the months of the year in reverse order, and subtraction of serial sevens from 100 (93, 86, 79 etc.).

(d) General information: choose questions appropriate to the patient's educational level. Suitable ones for average patients are the name of the monarch, Prime Minister, names of six large towns.

(e) Intelligence, as estimated by the interviewer.

Cognitive function should always be tested, as unsuspected defects which indicate organic cerebral dysfunction may be found.

7. *Insight into illness.*

Physical Examination

All inpatients should have a physical examination including a neurological one. Ideally outpatients should have one too, but in practice it is reserved for those in whom there is particular reason to suspect organic pathology.

Interview with Informant

A separate interview with an informant, usually the nearest relative, is essential if the patient is too disturbed or uncooperative to give a full history. It often adds useful information in other cases too, especially on the subject of premorbid personality, but should only be done with the patient's consent.

Formulation

The formulation is a critical summary of the case which should include both the positive features of the history and examination, and any relevant negative ones; differential diagnosis, with evidence for and against each possibility; the intended investigation, which may include a social worker's report, psychological testing, and laboratory tests; the plan for management, and comments on prognosis. There is no consensus of opinion on the correct length or content of a formulation; some psychiatrists interpret the term as a short list or summary of the relevant factors, others as a detailed discussion of the case which emphasizes its psychodynamic aspects.

Structured Interviews

Standardized interview schedules for research purposes have been developed from the history-taking scheme. The best known is the Present State Examination or PSE (Wing *et al.*, 1974). This is concerned only with symptoms and signs in the preceding month. There are some mandatory questions, but the interviewer may also inquire freely about areas which appear relevant. It has a high inter-rater reliability. The results can be processed by computer (CATEGO programme) to produce a diagnosis. Another semi-structured interview is the Standardized Psychiatric Interview (Goldberg *et al.*, 1970) which was developed for use in general practice and is largely concerned with neurotic symptoms.

Investigations

Since it may be impossible to distinguish between organic and functional psychiatric conditions by the history and mental state examination, all new patients should ideally have some laboratory investigations: blood count and ESR, urea and electrolytes, urine testing for glucose, protein, cells and bacteria, chest X-ray, thyroid function tests, and a WR. In practice these tests are routine for inpatients only. Blood and urine tests for drugs and alcohol should be done if abuse of these substances is suspected, and other specialized tests according to the clinical indications.

Psychological tests: psychometric tests alone are seldom diagnostic of organic impairment which is not clinically obvious, but they can provide evidence for or against its presence in doubtful cases. They are helpful in assessing the severity and location of the impairment in known cases, and repeated testing can be useful in monitoring progress. Tests used include those of intelligence, memory, perception, and ability for abstract thinking.

The electroencephalogram (EEG) may aid the diagnosis of focal lesions and of epilepsy, in which there is 'spike and wave' activity, 3/sec in petit mal and 4–8/sec in temporal lobe epilepsy. The EEG is usually abnormal in all disorders which cause organic cerebral dysfunction, although the type of abnormality is seldom specific for a particular disorder. The EEG can therefore help in diagnosing organic cases and in monitoring their progress.

Types of EEG activity include:

1. Alpha rhythm, 8–13 Hz (cycles/sec): recorded from the post-central region in most waking adults with the eyes closed, disappearing during mental activity or visual attention.
2. Beta rhythm, 13–30 Hz: recorded from the pre-central region in waking adults.
3. Theta rhythm, 4–7 Hz, and delta rhythm, less than 4 Hz: present in sleeping adults, and in infants and old people when awake.

Patients with functional psychiatric illness usually have a normal EEG. Sociopathic personality disorder is associated with an immature EEG pattern in 50% of cases. Psychotropic drugs usually alter the EEG; barbiturates and benzodiazepines increase fast activity, neuroleptics and tricyclic antidepressants produce slow waves and increase any epileptic activity. ECT produces slow waves which may persist for up to three months.

Brain scans: radioisotope scans are done by injecting a dose of technetium-99 or mercury-197 intravenously, then taking dynamic pictures as it circulates through the brain, and static pictures a few hours later. There is increased uptake of isotope in any abnormal area.

CT (computerized tomography) scans involve scanning from various angles using an X-ray rube and detector system, and reconstruction of cross-sectional or coronal pictures by computer.

Scans detect about 90% of lesions. CT scans are better than radio-isotope scans because they distinguish between types of lesion more clearly, can demonstrate the ventricular system, and are non-invasive.

Further Reading

Detailed accounts of history-taking and mental state examination are given in the short book by Leff and Isaacs (1978) and in the booklet published by the Institute of Psychiatry (1973). The investigation of organic cases is fully discussed in the book by Lishman (1978).

References

Goldberg, D. P., Cooper, B., Eastwood, M. R., Kedward, H. B., and Shepherd, M. (1970). A standardized psychiatric interview for use in community surveys. *Br. J. Prev. Soc. Med.* **24**, 18–23.
Institute of Psychiatry, Department of Psychiatry Teaching Committee (1973). *Notes on Eliciting and Recording Clinical Information.* Oxford University Press, London.

Leff, J. P., and Isaacs, A. D. (1978). *Psychiatric Examination in Clinical Practice*. Blackwell Scientific Publications, Oxford.

Lishman, W. A. (1978). *Organic Psychiatry*. Blackwell Scientific Publications, Oxford.

Wing, J. K., Cooper, J. E., and Sartorius, N. (1974). *The Measurement and Classification of Psychiatric Symptoms*. Cambridge University Press, Cambridge.

CHAPTER 3

Schizophrenia

Definition

The WHO definition of schizophrenic psychoses begins: 'A group of psychoses in which there is a fundamental disturbance of personality, a characteristic distortion of thinking, often a sense of being controlled by alien forces, delusions which may be bizarre, disturbed perception, abnormal affect out of keeping with the real situation, and autism. Nevertheless, clear consciousness and intellectual capacity are usually maintained' (World Health Organization, 1978).

Incidence and Prevalence

There are 20 new cases per 100,000 population per year, and the prevalence is 2–4 cases per 1000 population.

Epidemiology

1. *Age:* the commonest age of onset is late adolescence or early adult life.

2. *Sex:* slightly more men than women are affected.

3. *Marital status:* single status is more common than in the general population.

4. *Nationality:* the rates are similar in most countries, although apparent differences exist probably because of varying diagnostic criteria (World Health Organization, 1979). Immigrants have high rates.

5. *Social class:* highest rates in classes IV and V. This is the effect of 'drift down the social scale' in the early stages of the illness, not a result of being born into these classes.

6. *Premorbid personality:* of schizoid type (Chapter 6) in about 50% of cases.

Aetiology

1. *Genetics* (Gottesman and Shields, 1976): genetic predisposition to schizophrenia is proven. The observed familial pattern would fit with either polygenic inheritance, or a single gene of intermediate penetrance.

The expectation of developing schizophrenia before age 55 is 1% for the general population, and as follows among those related to a patient with schizophrenia:

Parent	6%
Sibling	10%
Child (one parent schizophrenic)	14%
Child (both parents schizophrenic)	46%

Concordance rates for schizophrenia in monozygotic twins are 35–58% and for dizygotic twins 9–26% in different series.

Similar rates are found among the relatives of schizophrenic patients even when they do not share the same environment, as shown by studies of children of schizophrenic mothers adopted in infancy, and of twins reared apart.

2. *Biochemistry:*

(a) Dopamine hypothesis (Crow *et al.*, 1976): this is the most widely accepted biochemical explanation for the 'positive' symptoms of acute schizophrenia. Dopamine is an inhibitory monoamine neurotransmitter, synthesized from L-tyrosine via L-dopa. Dopamine is concentrated in three areas of the brain: the nigrostriatal tract (dopamine depletion in this area results in Parkinsonism), the hypothalamus (inhibiting release of prolactin), and the mesolimbic system. The dopamine hypothesis states that schizophrenia results from excess dopamine activity in the mesolimbic system, which could be due to excess dopamine, deficiency of the dopamine antagonists gamma-aminobutyric acid (GABA) and acetylcholine, or increased sensitivity of dopamine receptors. The evidence in support of this theory includes the observations that neuroleptic drugs block dopamine receptors, and the capacity of individual drugs to do so correlates with their neuroleptic potency; that a schizophreniform psychosis may be precipitated by drugs which increase dopaminergic activity (amphetamines, LSD, atropine, L-dopa); and that post-mortem studies have shown either excess dopamine concentration in the mesolimbic system, or proliferation of dopamine receptors there, in brains from schizophrenic patients.

(b) Aberrant methylation hypothesis: this states that schizophrenic symptoms result from methylation of amine neurotransmitters. The theory came into fashion after the finding of a 'pink spot', thought to be due to excretion of dimethoxyphenylethylamine (DMPE) which is a methylated derivative of dopamine, on chromatography of patients' urine. The 'pink spot' was probably an artefact, but there is some evidence that the hallucinogen dimethyltryptamine (DMT) is excreted by schizophrenic patients, and the symptoms of schizophrenia may be exacerbated by methionine which is a methyl group donor.

(c) Endorphin abnormality: endorphins are brain peptides which bind to the same receptors as opiates do. They are concerned with the perception of pain, which may be either increased or decreased in schizophrenia. Naloxone is a drug which blocks these receptors, and it has been reported to stop hallucinations in schizophrenia.

(d) Prostaglandin abnormality.

(e) Virus-like agents have been reported in the CSF of some schizophrenic patients.

Other biological observations of unknown significance have been made, including lowered reactivity of the autonomic nervous system, resistance to the effects of drugs, nitrogen retention in periodic catatonia, minor EEG abnormalities, cerebral atrophy in chronic cases, abnormalities of cerebral lateralization, abnormal eye movements, low platelet monoamine oxidase (MAO), an association with temporal lobe epilepsy of the dominant hemisphere, and an excess of winter births.

3. *Psychological theories:*

(a) Abnormal concept formation may be the cause of schizophrenic thought disorder. Concepts are inconsistent and overinclusive, and abstract concepts cannot be formed.

(b) The 'sensory filter' which limits the amount of sensory information reaching consciousness is defective, so that patients are overstimulated by their environment, and unable to direct their attention selectively.

4. *Psychodynamic theories:* it has been postulated that schizophrenia develops as a reaction to, or defence against, abnormal communications within the family (Lidz, 1968). The features described in schizophrenic

patients' families include an overprotective yet hostile mother; a distorted relationship ('schism' or 'skew') between the mother and father; and the 'double-bind' (Bateson *et al.*, 1956) in which the mother's communications to the child are inconsistent, e.g. affectionate words accompanied by rejecting behaviour. Such observations have not been reproduced in later investigations, and it is possible that any abnormalities of family interaction are a secondary effect of a schizophrenic illness in one or more members, rather than being of aetiological importance.

However, it is established that psychological stress can influence the course of schizophrenia. An increased frequency of life events (Chapter 23) has been found during the three weeks prior to a schizophrenic breakdown (Brown and Birley, 1968). High levels of critical 'expressed emotion' shown towards patients by their relatives predispose to relapse (Brown *et al.*, 1972; Vaughn and Leff, 1976).

Clinical Features

Onset of the illness may be sudden or gradual. The symptoms may include abnormalities of thought, ideation (i.e. delusions), perception (i.e. hallucinations), emotion, volition, or motor behaviour.

Thought: 'thought interference' is a feeling that thoughts are being withdrawn, inserted, or broadcast by an external agent. 'Thought block' is the abrupt cessation of a train of thought. 'Derailment of thought', 'knight's move thinking' or 'asyndetic thinking' is a loss of logical connection between one thought sequence and the next, causing incomprehensible shifts in topic. 'Nebulosity' of thought is inability to focus on the point without being diverted by irrelevant side issues. 'Concrete thought' is inability to appreciate abstract concepts; although some patients assume symbolic meanings when they are not intended. The abnormalities of thought are reflected in speech, which ranges from vague and difficult to follow, to incomprehensibly bizarre. Severely thought-disordered patients may speak in a jumble of words ('word salad') and include their own idiosyncratic words (neologisms).

Delusions may be preceded by 'delusional mood' in which the patient feels perplexed by a feeling that the surrounding environment has changed in a strange way. This feeling is followed by the sudden appearance of a 'primary (autochthonous) delusion', usually in association with an ordinary perception ('delusional perception'). Delusions are most commonly paranoid but may be of other types. A complex system of secondary delusions may be elaborated from the primary one.

Hallucinations are most commonly auditory, typically voices discussing the patient in the third person. The patient attributes them to an external source. Somatic, tactile, olfactory, or gustatory hallucinations may also occur, but visual ones are unusual.

Emotion: the most typical emotional change is that of 'blunting (or flattening) of affect', in which the patient shows very little emotion. 'Incongruity of affect' is demonstration of an emotion which is inappropriate to the circumstances. Extreme emotional changes of elation, depression or rage may occur.

Volition: passivity feelings, in which the patient feels that his emotions or actions are being controlled by an outside agent, may be present. Most patients lack initiative and drive.

Motor behaviour: abnormalities include mannerisms, stereotypies, imitation of the speech and behaviour of others, negativism, mutism, stupor, hyperkinesis, and prolonged maintenance of strange postures.

Intellectual function: it was once believed that formal intellectual defects did not occur, but they are demonstrable in many chronic schizophrenics (Owens and Johnstone, 1980).

Clinical Types (World Health Organization 1978)

The following types are described in the ICD, but there is overlap between them as regards symptoms and prognosis.

Simple schizophrenia is characterized by the 'negative' symptoms of gradual deterioration of the personality, with flattening of affect, withdrawal from reality, and loss of drive, resulting in a life-style of social isolation and self-neglect. 'Positive' symptoms like delusions and hallucinations do not occur, and therefore it is debatable whether a diagnosis of schizophrenia is appropriate in such cases.

Hebephrenic schizophrenia has an acute onset and florid symptoms which usually include delusions and hallucinations, thought disorder, and affective changes.

Catatonic schizophrenia, which is rare, has predominantly motor symptoms.

Paranoid schizophrenia has delusions, which are often accompanied by hallucinations, as the most prominent symptom. The general personality may be quite well preserved, in which case the condition may be called 'paraphrenia'. Paranoid schizophrenia usually develops later in life than the other types and schizophrenia starting after middle age nearly always takes this form. It is commoner in women. Impaired hearing is present in about 40% of patients, and there is also an increased prevalence of visual impairment.

Acute schizophrenic episode (oneirophrenia) includes a dream-like clouding of consciousness as well as schizophrenic symptoms. Such episodes may remit without treatment.

Latent schizophrenia (borderline schizophrenia, pseudoneurotic schizophrenia) is a vague term sometimes applied to patients who give an impression of being schizophrenic but have no definite symptoms.

Residual schizophrenia is the 'defect state' which may remain following an acute episode. Positive symptoms have faded but there is blunting of affect and thought disorder.

Schizoaffective psychosis (cycloid psychosis) is a condition in which manic or depressive symptoms coexist with schizophrenic ones. There are remissions and relapses, as in the affective psychoses.

Diagnostic Criteria

There is no universal agreement about which illnesses should be classified as 'schizophrenia' (Kendell, 1972). Problems include:

1. whether the term should be reserved for illnesses which result in permanent defects in personality (nuclear or process schizophrenia), or also used for acute episodes (schizophreniform reactions) which may recover completely.
2. whether there is a valid distinction between schizophrenia and the affective psychoses.

When Kraepelin described the condition in 1898 under the name 'dementia praecox' he distinguished it from manic-depressive illness because of its worse prognosis. E. Bleuler, who gave it the name 'schizophrenia' (Bleuler, 1911), considered that its essential features were loosening of associations in thought, flattening or incongruity of affect, ambivalence, and autism (withdrawal from reality), and that it always led to some defect in personality. As these symptoms cannot be clearly defined, widely differing concepts of 'schizophrenia' developed in different centres, for example schizophrenia was diagnosed more readily in the USA than in the UK.

In recent years there have been attempts to standardize the definition using reliable diagnostic criteria. The most widely used system in Britain is that of Schneider (1959), who postulated a set of 'first rank symptoms', any one of which should be considered diagnostic of schizophrenia in the absence of organic brain disease. They are:

1. Auditory hallucinations in one of three forms: voices discussing the patient in the third person, voices making a running commentary on his actions, and voices repeating his thoughts aloud (*echo de la pensée*).
2. Thought insertion, withdrawal, or broadcasting (thought interference).
3. Passivity feelings.
4. Primary delusions.

Schneider's criteria are arbitrary, do not predict long-term outcome, and may occur in patients who have affective psychoses rather than schizophrenia.

Many other sets of diagnostic criteria have been proposed. There is poor concordance between them (Brockington *et al.*, 1978).

Differential Diagnosis

1. Organic brain disease.
2. Drug-induced psychosis (LSD and amphetamines being the commonest drugs concerned).
3. Affective disorder.
4. Personality disorder.
5. Acute reactions to stress, especially in adolescence.
6. Simulation of mental illness.

Some of these conditions may present in a way which is indistinguishable from schizophrenia, and the correct diagnosis requires investigation and a period of observation.

Treatment

1. *Drugs:* neuroleptic drugs (Chapter 20) are effective in about 90% of cases. 'Positive' symptoms respond to drugs better than 'negative' ones. Treatment may need to be continued for up to four weeks before improvement occurs. Chlorpromazine, 500–1000 mg daily in divided doses, is usually used. In theory, all the neuroleptic drugs should be equally effective although some may prove better than others in an individual patient. There is a widely held belief that trifluoperazine is the best drug for treating delusions.

The efficacy of neuroleptics in treating acute schizophrenia is well established, but their place in maintenance treatment is less clear. Patients judged to have a bad prognosis (see below) are usually kept on neuroleptics indefinitely, and those judged to have a good prognosis may have the drugs withdrawn a few months after recovery. Patients in the intermediate prognosis group are less likely to relapse if maintained on neuroleptics (Leff and Wing, 1971), but some patients of this kind may not need them. As long-term therapy carries a high risk of side-effects, and wastes time and money if not necessary, it is worth stopping the drugs in the intermediate prognosis group to see whether relapse occurs or not.

Long-term neuroleptics are usually given by intramuscular depot injections. This method improves compliance with medication, as many schizophrenic patients are unreliable about taking tablets. It also means that patients are seen regularly by the community nurse or GP.

Propranolol in high dose has been reported to have a beneficial effect in schizophrenia (Yorkston *et al.*, 1977), but requires further evaluation.

2. *ECT* (Chapter 21) has not been formally evaluated as a sole treatment for schizophrenia, but clinical experience suggests that it is often effective for patients who have failed to respond to neuroleptics, who have a depressive component to their illness, or have catatonic symptoms.

3. *Social aspects:* most new cases start treatment as inpatients. Following control of the acute symptoms, it is generally useful for them to have some months' rehabilitation as inpatients or day patients. They are often handicapped by slowness, unreliability, lack of initiative, social withdrawal, and poor self-care. They may improve with tuition in work, personal care, practical aspects of daily living, and social skills, but many never recover their premorbid level of functioning.

A patient who has had a schizophrenic illness requires some degree of support and guidance, but excessive stimulation predisposes to relapse. A family in which other members focus much emotion or criticism towards the patient is not desirable (Vaughn and Leff, 1976), and a hostel or group home may provide a more suitable environment.

Prognosis

Between 25% and 50% of patients make a good recovery, about 25% remain severely handicapped, and the rest are able to live independently but have obvious residual defects. The most common residual problems are slowness, withdrawal, unreliability, and lack of initiative, which in hospitalized patients could be due to institutionalization as well as the illness itself (Wing and Brown, 1970).

Poor prognostic features (Editorial, 1977) are a positive family history, schizoid premorbid personality, low IQ, low social class, single or divorced status, asthenic build, and an illness beginning in early life, with gradual onset, no precipitating factors, lack of insight, impaired abstract thought, apathy, affective flattening, and paranoid delusions.

Up to 15% of deaths among schizophrenics result from suicide.

Further Reading

A detailed account of schizophrenia and its management is given in the book edited by Wing (1978).

References

Bateson, G., Jackson, D. D., Haley, J., and Weakland, J. H. (1956). Toward a theory of schizophrenia. *Behav. Sci.*, **1**, 251–264.

Bleuler, E. (1911). *Dementia Praecox or the Group of Schizophrenias.* Trans. J. Zinkin, 1950. International Universities Press, New York.

Brockington, I. F., Kendell, R. E., and Leff, J. P. (1978). Definitions of schizophrenia: concordance and prediction of outcome. *Psychol. Med.*, **8**, 387–398.

Brown, G. W., and Birley, J. L. T. (1968). Crises and life changes and the onset of schizophrenia. *J. Health Soc. Behav.*, **9**, 203–214.

Brown, G. W., Birley, J. L. T., and Wing, J. K. (1972). Influence of family life on the course of schizophrenic disorders: a replication. *Br. J. Psychiatry*, **121**, 241–258.

Crow, T. J., Deakin, J. F. W., Johnstone, E. C., and Longden, A. (1976). Dopamine and schizophrenia. *Lancet*, **ii**, 563–566.

Editorial (1977). First attacks of schizophrenia. *Br. Med. J.*, **1**, 733–734.

Gottesman, I. I., and Shields, J. (1976). Critical review of recent adoption, twin and family studies. *Schizophr. Bull.*, **2**, 360–400.

Kendell, R. E. (1972). Schizophrenia: the remedy for diagnostic confusion. *Br. J. Hosp. Med.*, **8**, 383–390.

Leff, J. P., and Wing, J. K. (1971). Trial of maintenance therapy in schizophrenia. *Br. Med. J.*, 3, 599–604.

Lidz, T. (1968). The family, language and transmission of schizophrenia. In *The Transmission of Schizophrenia* (Eds. D. Rosenthal and S. Kety). Pergamon Press, Oxford.

Owens, D. G. C., and Johnstone, E. C. (1980). The disabilities of chronic schizophrenia — their nature and the factors contributing to their development. *Br. J. Psychiatry* 136, 384–395.

Schneider, K. (1959). *Clinical Psychopathology*. Trans. M. W. Hamilton. Grune and Stratton, New York.

Vaughn, C. E. and Leff, J. P. (1976). The influence of family and social factors on the course of psychiatric illness. *Br. J. Psychiatry* 129, 125–137.

Wing, J. K. (Ed.) (1978). *Schizophrenia: Towards a New Synthesis*. Academic Press, London.

Wing, J. K., and Brown, G. W. (1970). *Institutionalism and Schizophrenia*. Cambridge University Press, Cambridge.

World Health Organization (1978). *Mental Disorders: Glossary and Guide to their Classification in Accordance with the Ninth Revision of the International Classification of Diseases*. WHO, Geneva.

World Health Organization (1979). *Schizophrenia: an International Follow-up Study*. Wiley, Chichester.

Yorkston, N. J., Gruzelier, J. H., Zaki, S. A., Hollander, D., Pitcher, D. R., and Sergeant, H. G. S. (1977). Propranolol as an adjunct to the treatment of schizophrenia. *Lancet* ii, 575–578.

CHAPTER 4

Affective Disorders

Definition

Affective disorders are conditions in which the primary disturbance is a change of mood. They include depressive illness and mania.

Classification

Patients with episodes of both depression and mania are said to have 'bipolar affective disorder' (manic depressive psychosis), and those with episodes of depression only to have 'unipolar affective disorder'. Patients with mania are assumed to have bipolar affective disorder, since virtually all of them will have episodes of depression too if they live long enough.

Depressive illness can be divided into 'depressive neurosis' and 'depressive psychosis'. These terms are roughly equivalent to the older ones 'reactive depression' and 'endogenous depression'. It is not clear whether they are two distinct conditions, or whether their characteristic symptom clusters represent the extreme ends of a continuous spectrum in which most patients are intermediate between the two (Kendell, 1976).

Incidence and Prevalence

The lifetime expectancy of being admitted to hospital for affective disorder is 2% for men and 4% for women. Affective disorders of lesser severity are much more common, but their reported frequency varies in different prevalence studies because there can be no agreed boundary between mild depressive illness and 'normal' unhappiness. The prevalence of depressive illness in the general population is probably about 4%, depressive neurosis being at least twice as common as depressive psychosis, and mania much less frequent.

Epidemiology

1. *Age:* episodes may occur at any age including childhood, but depressive neurosis most commonly affects young adults whereas depressive psychosis and mania both become more frequent with increasing age.

2. *Sex:* twice as common in women.

3. *Premorbid personality* (Chodoff, 1972): typically asthenic for depressive neurosis, stable for depressive psychosis, and cyclothymic for manic-depressive psychosis, but exceptions are frequent.

Aetiology

1. *Genetics* (Reveley and Murray, 1980): genetic predisposition is proven, but it is not clear whether a single gene with incomplete penetrance, polygenic inheritance, or an X-linked gene is responsible. First degree relatives of patients with affective disorder have a 10–15% chance of developing it themselves. Concordance rates are 68% for monozygotic twins and 23% for dizygotic ones. Unipolar and bipolar affective disorders appear genetically distinct from one another, but depressive neurosis and depressive psychosis do not.

2. *Biochemistry:*

(a) Monoamine neurotransmitters: brain concentrations of noradrenaline (NA) or 5-hydroxytryptamine (5-HT) or both are thought to be reduced in depressive illness, whereas concentrations of dopamine and perhaps other neurotransmitters are increased in mania. The evidence for this includes the observations that antidepressant drugs increase brain monoamine concentrations; hypotensive drugs, e.g. reserpine, which deplete monoamine concentrations may cause depression; neuroleptic drugs block dopamine receptors and have a therapeutic effect in mania; plasma tryptophan, a precursor of 5-HT, is reduced in some depressives; and concentrations of 5-HT and its metabolite 5-hydroxyindole acetic acid (5-HIAA) are reduced in the brains of some depressed patients who have committed suicide. However, excretion of monoamine metabolites is not consistently low in depressives; and neither L-dopa, precursor of dopamine and noradrenaline, nor L-tryptophan is effective for treating depression. These studies are difficult because minor concentrations are involved, concentrations of metabolites may reflect changes in peripheral rather than central monoamines, and findings can be affected by diet, exercise and non-specific stress.

(b) Electrolytes: intracellular sodium is increased in depressive illness, and further increased in mania.

(c) Endocrines: in depressive illness, cortisol secretion is approximately doubled, its diurnal variation is absent, and it is not suppressed by dexamethasone. TSH secretion is reduced and glucose tolerance is reduced.

3. *Sociology:* life events during the months preceding the onset of depressive illness occur with higher than expected frequency (Paykel *et al.*, 1969). Undesirable events, especially those involving loss, account for the excess. The finding applies to both depressive neurosis and depressive psychosis. There is also some evidence that a less recent event, death of the mother in childhood, predisposes to depressive illness (Tennant *et al.*, 1980). These observations are consistent with the psycho-analytic theory that depression results from internalized aggression, following identification with a lost love object.

Depressive neurosis in London working class women has been found to correlate with a poor marital relationship, having three or more young children at home, and absence of outside employment (Brown *et al.*, 1975).

4. *Behavioural theories:* depression can be considered as a state of low self-esteem, or 'learned helplessness' (Seligman, 1972), developed following repeated failure to overcome problems by personal effort. Once acquired, depressive symptoms may continue because they evoke attention and sympathy.

Clinical Features

Depressive psychosis: most patients feel depressed in mood, but some complain of a lack of feeling instead. Some are agitated, others retarded. Feelings of guilt, unworthiness, and hopelessness, leading to suicidal thoughts or acts, are frequent. Biological symptoms include early morning waking, diurnal variation in mood with improvement as the day progresses, anorexia, weight loss, constipation, and loss of libido which may be accompanied by amenorrhoea or impotence. Interest and concentration are reduced and memory impaired, probably because of concentration difficulties. Physical complaints, e.g. headache, backache, and facial pain, are prominent in some patients. Severe cases may have delusions, with paranoid, hypochondriacal or nihilistic content (Cotard's syndrome), and hallucinations, typically voices which address the patient in critical terms. Obsessional or hysterical features may be present. 'Involutional melancholia' is an agitated depressive illness which starts in later life.

Depressive neurosis: symptoms may be seen as an exaggeration of understandable unhappiness, arising in response to stress, and often mixed with anxiety. Biological symptoms are not severe, and delusions and hallucinations do not occur. There is difficulty getting off to sleep, rather than early morning waking; fluctuation of mood according to circumstances, rather than regular diurnal variation; self-pity rather than guilt.

A diagnosis of depressive illness may be made when depressed mood is inappropriately severe or prolonged in relation to its cause, or is accompanied by characteristic biological symptoms and changes in attitude. Scales used to measure its severity include the Hamilton Rating Scale (Hamilton, 1967), Beck Depression Inventory (Beck *et al.*, 1961), and Zung Self Rating Depression Scale (Zung, 1965).

Mania: elation of mood is the essential feature, and may be manifest as cheerfulness, irritability, or aggression. Energy is increased, with over-activity, disinhibition, distractibility, reduced need for food and sleep, increased sexual interest, and financial extravagance. This behaviour may have very unfortunate consequences for the patient and others. Thought and speech are rapid and copious ('pressure of speech'), often with loose connections between one subject and the next ('flight of ideas'), rhymes, and puns. Thought content is usually grandiose, sometimes paranoid. There may be delusions and hallucinations, also with a grandiose or paranoid content. 'Manic stupor' is a rare form in which activity is greatly reduced, despite an elated mood and grandiose thought content. 'Hypomania' is a mild form of mania. Transient periods of depression occur during the course of most manic illnesses, and if these are prominent, the condition may be called a 'mixed affective state'.

Natural History (Winokur and Morrison, 1973)

Most episodes of affective illness remit within a few months even without treatment, and patients remain quite well between episodes. Less often a single episode becomes chronic and lasts for years, or episodes are so frequent that there is no intervening period of normality. Bipolar patients may alternate between depressed and manic phases, or one or other phase may predominate. Some patients become ill with a regular frequency, or at a certain time of year, usually spring or autumn. However, the course in any individual patient is unpredictable. 10–15% of patients die by suicide.

Differential Diagnosis of Depressive Illness

1. *Physical conditions:* depressed mood is a frequent symptom of certain diseases including hypothyroidism, Parkinson's disease, senile and arteriosclerotic dementia, B_{12} deficiency, and multiple sclerosis, and may follow virus infections such as influenza and hepatitis. Drugs which can cause depression include hypotensives, especially reserpine and methyldopa, neuroleptics, steroids, the contraceptive pill, digitalis, L-dopa, and sulphonamides.

2. *Psychiatric conditions:* depressed mood can accompany most psychiatric illnesses, and it is often difficult to determine whether depressive illness is the primary condition; this is particularly so when depression is mixed with anxiety, and in 'schizoaffective' states.

Differential Diagnosis of Mania

1. *Physical conditions:* frontal lobe lesions, Cushing's syndrome, multiple sclerosis, and drugs including steroids, amphetamines, L-dopa, and antidepressants may produce euphoria.

2. *Psychiatric conditions:* elated mood may occur in schizophrenia, and disinhibited behaviour similar to that of hypomania may occur with personality disorders.

Treatment of Depressive Illness (Shaw, 1977)

Severely depressed patients require hospital admission if they are refusing food and drink, are suicidal, or as occasionally happens are homicidal.

1. *Drugs* (Chapter 20): a tricyclic antidepressant, or one of the newer related drugs, is usually chosen as the first line of treatment. It may take

three weeks to work. If effective, it should be continued for at least six months to reduce the risk of relapse (Mindham *et al.*, 1973). Tricyclics are effective in about 70% of depressed patients (MRC, 1965) and work better in depressive psychosis than depressive neurosis (Kiloh *et al.*, 1962).

Monoamine oxidase inhibitors (MAOIs) are used mainly for depressive neurosis, especially when anxiety is prominent. They are usually ineffective in depressive psychosis (MRC, 1965). The combination of a MAOI and a tricyclic, sometimes used for resistant cases, has no advantage over a single drug for routine use (Young *et al.*, 1979).

Other drugs with antidepressant activity are flupenthixol, a neuroleptic, and the amino acid tryptophan. Phenothiazines are a useful adjunct to other treatments in the agitated or deluded patient. Lithium may be useful in treating depression, as well as in preventing it, but requires more evaluation (Mendels, 1976).

2. *ECT* (Chapter 21): ECT works more quickly than drugs and is therefore the treatment of choice for severely depressed patients. It is effective in at least 80% of patients with depressive psychosis (MRC, 1965), but less effective in depressive neurosis. It is better than tricyclics if delusions are present. It is also used if drugs have failed, or if medical contraindications to tricyclics are present. Antidepressants combined with ECT, and continued at least six months afterwards, reduce the risk of relapse and may reduce the number of treatments required in the ECT course.

3. *Psychotherapy* (Chapter 22): there is some evidence that psychotherapy, alone or combined with drugs, is effective in depressive neurosis (Weissman, 1979). Intensive psychotherapy is generally considered inappropriate in depressive psychosis, as it may increase patients' feelings of guilt and unworthiness, and will not affect delusions or hallucinations.

4. *Leucotomy* (Chapter 21): leucotomy is only used for severe long-standing cases which have failed to respond to other treatments. It has a success rate of about 70%.

Treatment of Mania

Hospital admission is desirable to prevent the adverse consequences of extravagance and disinhibited behaviour. Drugs are the first line of treatment and either neuroleptics or lithium are effective. Lithium takes about a week to act and so is most suitable for mild cases; it is the best drug for mixed affective states. If drugs have failed to control a manic illness, a few ECT treatments often succeed.

Prophylaxis of Affective Disorder (Quitkin *et al.*, 1976)

Lithium is an effective prophylactic. It works better in bipolar than in unipolar disease. As lithium prophylaxis involves regular medication and follow-up and may cause side-effects, it is only justified when episodes of illness are frequent and severe; at least three attacks in two years is a rough guide. Long-term antidepressant medication is an alternative prophylactic in unipolar patients, as is 'maintenance' ECT at monthly intervals although this has not been formally evaluated.

Further Reading

A detailed account of affective disorders and their treatment is given in the books edited by Paykel and Coppen (1979) and by Coppen and Walk (1968).

References

Beck, A. T., Ward, C. H., Mendelson, M., Mock, J., and Erbaugh, J. (1961). An inventory for measuring depression. *Arch. Gen. Psychiatry* **4**, 561–571.

Brown, G. W., Bhrolchain, M. N., and Harris, T. (1975). Social class and psychiatric disturbance among women in an urban population. *Sociology* **9**, 225–254.

Chodoff, P. (1972). The depressive personality: a critical review. *Arch. Gen. Psychiatry* **27**, 666–673.

Coppen, A., and Walk, A. (Eds.) (1968). *Recent Developments in Affective Disorders*. Headley Bros., Ashford, Kent.

Hamilton, M. (1967). Development of a rating scale for primary depressive illness. *Br. J. Soc. Clin. Psychol.* **6**, 278–296.

Kendell, R. E. (1976). The classification of depressions: a review of contemporary confusion. *Br. J. Psychiatry* **129**, 15–28.

Kiloh, L., Ball, J. R. B., and Garside, R. F. (1962). Prognostic factors in treatment of depressive states with imipramine. *Br. Med. J.* **1**, 1225–1227.

Medical Research Council (1965). Clinical trial of the treatment of depressive illness. *Br. Med. J.* **1**, 881–886.

28

Mendels, J. (1976). Lithium in the treatment of depression. *Am. J. Psychiatry* **133**, 373-378.

Mindham, R. H. S., Howland, C., and Shepherd, M. (1973). An evaluation of continuation therapy with tricyclic antidepressants in depressive illness. *Psychol. Med.* **3**, 5-17.

Paykel, E. S., and Coppen, A. (Eds.) (1979). *Psychopharmacology of Affective Disorders.* Oxford University Press, Oxford.

Paykel, E. S., Myers, J. K., Dienelt, M. N., Klerman, G. L., Lindenthal, J. J., and Pepper, M. P. (1969). Life events and depression. *Arch. Gen. Psychiatry,* **21**, 753-760.

Quitkin, F., Rifkin, A., and Klein, D. F. (1976). Prophylaxis of affective disorders: current status of knowledge. *Arch. Gen. Psychiatry,* **33**, 337-341.

Reveley, A., and Murray, R. M. (1980). The genetic contribution to the functional psychoses. *Br. J. Hosp. Med.,* **24**, 166-171.

Seligman, M. E. P. (1972). Learned helplessness. *Annu. Rev. Med.* **23**, 407-412.

Shaw, D. (1977). Review article: the practical management of affective disorders. *Br. J. Psychiatry* **130**, 432-451.

Tennant, C., Bebbington, P., and Hurry, J. (1980). Parental death in childhood and risk of adult depressive disorders: a review. *Psychol. Med.* **10**, 289-299.

Weissman, M. M. (1979). The psychological treatment of depression. *Arch. Gen. Psychiatry* **36**, 1261-1269.

Winokur, G., and Morrison, J. (1973). The Iowa 500: follow-up of 225 depressives. *Br. J. Psychiatry* **123**, 543-548.

Young, J. P. R., Lader, M. H., and Hughes, W. C. (1979). Controlled trial of imipramine, monoamine oxidase inhibitors, and combined treatment in depressed outpatients. *Br. Med. J.* **2**, 1315-1318.

Zung, W. (1965). A self-rating depression scale. *Arch. Gen. Psychiatry* **12**, 63-70.

CHAPTER 5

Neuroses

WHO definition: 'Neurotic disorders are mental disorders without any demonstrable organic basis in which the patient may have considerable insight and has unimpaired reality testing, in that he usually does not confuse his morbid subjective experiences and fantasies with external reality. Behaviour may be greatly affected although usually remaining within socially acceptable limits, but personality is not disorganised. The principal manifestations include excessive anxiety, hysterical symptoms, phobias, obsessional and compulsive symptoms, and depression' (World Health Organization, 1978).

Prevalence

Community surveys show that about 10% of the population are affected by neurotic symptoms at any one time. An exact prevalence is impossible to determine as neurotic symptoms are not qualitatively different from normal experience.

Epidemiology

1. *Age:* neuroses usually start in early adult life.

2. *Sex:* women are affected twice as often as men.

3. *Premorbid personality:* neurotic tendencies have often been present since childhood.

Aetiology

1. *Genetics* (Murray and Reveley, 1981): a genetic predisposition is thought to exist because up to 20% of patients' first degree relatives are affected, usually by the same type of neurosis, and there is a higher

concordance for neurosis in monozygotic than dizygotic twins. Learning neurotic behaviour patterns in childhood, however, may partly account for the familial tendency.

2. *Environmental stress* can usually be identified as a precipitating factor.

Treatment

1. *Drugs* (Chapter 20): drugs are useful for the short-term treatment of acute episodes, but patients with chronic neurosis often become dependent on hypnotics or tranquillizers without deriving real benefit from their continued use.

2. *Psychotherapy* (Chapter 22): supportive psychotherapy and simple counselling are thought to be beneficial for most patients and their relatives. Patients with insight and motivation may improve after dynamic psychotherapy, individual or group, designed to explore the origins of their symptoms and change their ways of coping with life.

3. *Behaviour therapy* (Chapter 22): this is the treatment of choice for phobias and obsessions. Patients with other types of neurotic symptom often benefit from relaxation training, and social skills training.

4. *Social management:* environmental problems which are causing continued stress can sometimes be ameliorated by social casework, or the patient can be advised how to approach them more constructively. However, many of the common perpetuating stresses, e.g. an unhappy marriage, job dissatisfaction, poverty, are irremediable. In some cases they are a result of the neurosis, not its cause.

Prognosis

Some patients have a single episode which recovers completely, some have recurrent episodes, and others are chronically affected and incapacitated. Patients who develop an acute neurotic illness following temporary stress but had an adequate premorbid personality usually do well, whereas those with chronic symptoms, continuing life stress, and neurotic personality traits usually do badly, and have an increased risk of suicide.

The individual neuroses are described separately below, except for depressive neurosis which is included in the chapter on affective disorders (Chapter 4). Symptoms of more than one type may coexist in the same patient.

ANXIETY NEUROSIS (ANXIETY STATE) (Marks and Lader, 1973)

Definition

Anxiety has two components: an unpleasant mood characterized by uncertainty and fear, and physical symptoms most of which result from overactivity of the sympathetic nervous system. Anxiety neurosis is diagnosed when anxiety develops without an adequate cause, and it includes 'free-floating' and 'phobic' types.

Prevalence

5% of the population.

Epidemiology and Aetiology

As for neuroses in general.

Clinical Features

Mental symptoms are apprehension, poor concentration, worry, difficulty in getting off to sleep, and depersonalization. Physical symptoms are tachycardia, palpitations, chest pain, dyspnoea, nausea, anorexia, diarrhoea, fatigue, dizziness, sweating, tremor, headache, a 'lump in the throat', weakness of the legs, frequency of micturition, dry mouth, and flushing of the face and chest. Most patients have both mental and physical symptoms. 'Panic attacks' are episodes of acute anxiety with overbreathing which may lead to tetany or loss of consciousness. Symptoms of depressive neurosis are often mixed with those of anxiety neurosis.

Secretion of catecholamines, cortisol, and thyroid hormones is increased.

Phobic anxiety state (Marks, 1969) is a term used when the anxiety is aroused only by certain objects or situations, as opposed to being present continuously as in the 'free-floating' type of anxiety state. Examples of phobic stimuli are insects, animals, air travel, and eating in public. Sometimes these have been associated with an unpleasant experience in the past, in which case the phobia may be called a 'maladaptive learned response'. The anxiety may be confined to one particular object or situation ('monophobia') or may be associated with several stimuli and some free-floating anxiety. The patient's life may become dominated by avoidance of the phobic stimulus.

Agoraphobia ('house-bound housewife' or 'anxiety–depersonalization syndrome') consists of a fear of leaving the home, entering shops, or using public transport, especially if alone. Panic attacks are frequent if the patient enters the feared situation. Most patients are young married women of dependent personality, whose husbands are often over-protective towards them and have neurotic symptoms themselves.

Measurement of Anxiety

Measurements are of value in monitoring response to treatment, rather than in diagnosis. Psychological rating scales include the Taylor Manifest Anxiety Scale (Taylor, 1953), and line scales made for individual patients. Physiological measurements of sympathetic nervous system activity can also be used as an indication of change in the same subject on different occasions. They include galvanic skin response (GSR), pulse rate, blood pressure, forearm blood flow, salivary gland secretion, pupillography, electromyography, tremor measurement, eyeblink rate, EEG, and respiratory rate. These are non-specific indicators of arousal, whether in anxiety or other excited states, and their resting values vary between subjects.

Differential Diagnosis

1. *'Normal' anxiety:* some anxiety is to be expected in stressful situations, and does not require treatment unless it is so severe as to impair performance.

2. *Anxious personality:* it can be impossible to separate this from anxiety neurosis as the two often coexist.

3. *Psychiatric illness:* anxiety may be a symptom of another psychiatric condition such as depressive illness, schizophrenia, obsessional neurosis, dementia, and drug or alcohol withdrawal states.

4. *Physical illness:* thyrotoxicosis, phaeochromocytoma, paroxysmal tachycardia.

Other psychiatric or physical illness should be sought if anxiety symptoms first start in middle or old age.

Treatment

1. *Drugs:* anxiolytic drugs are best taken when symptoms occur, rather than in fixed dosage, to avoid tolerance or dependence. Benzodiazepines are the most widely used drugs. Beta blockers such as propranolol are useful if physical symptoms predominate. MAOIs are appropriate if depressive or phobic symptoms are present. Neuroleptics in low dose are effective and less likely than benzodiazepines to cause dependence, but because of their potential side-effects are not the drugs of first choice.

2. *Behaviour therapy:* this is the treatment of choice for phobic anxiety, in which systematic desensitization, modelling, or flooding may be used. Monophobias respond best. Relaxation training and biofeedback may be useful for control of physical symptoms. Social skills training is helpful for anxiety related to social interactions.

3. *Psychotherapy:* indicated where complex underlying problems appear to be contributing to the anxiety. Group therapy is suitable if interpersonal relationships are a source of difficulty.

4. *Leucotomy:* this is reserved for very severe intractable cases, and has a success rate of about 60%.

Prognosis

Prognosis is good when an anxiety state develops following a defined stress in someone of adequate premorbid personality, but poor when there are continuing stresses and inadequate personality.

OBSESSIVE–COMPULSIVE NEUROSIS (Beech, 1974)

Definition

A recurrent thought, image, feeling, impulse or movement, which the patient recognizes as being absurd and originating within his own mind, and resists without success.

Prevalence

0.05% of the population.

Epidemiology and Aetiology

1. *Age:* onset is usually in early adult life.

2. *Sex:* equal sex incidence.

3. *Premorbid personality:* usually anancastic (Chapter 6).

4. *Genetics:* about 5% of patients' first degree relatives are affected, and several pairs of monozygotic twins concordant for obsessive-compulsive neurosis have been found.

5. *Intelligence:* often above average.

6. *Brain damage* is sometimes present; encephalitis lethargica is especially likely to have obsessive-compulsive sequelae. Resistance to the symptoms is often absent in brain-damaged patients.

Clinical Features

Obsessive-compulsive phenomena include:

1. *Fears*, e.g. of harming others (which are never put into practice), or contracting a particular disease.

2. *Thoughts*, e.g. sexual or blasphemous ones which are abhorrent to the patient.

3. *Ruminations*, e.g. insoluble problems in mathematics or philosophy.

4. *Rituals*, e.g. checking or washing, often carried out in order to allay obsessional fears.

Patients know that their symptoms are absurd but they cannot overcome them unaided. They may spend so much time on their rituals that there is none left for daily life. The illness is very distressing both for the patients and for their relatives.

Differential Diagnosis

1. *Depressive illness* may give rise to obsessive-compulsive symptoms.

2. *Delusions, thought interference, and passivity experiences* can be distinguished from obsessional thoughts because the latter are recognized by the patient as being abnormal and originating in his own mind.

3. *Stereotyped behaviour* in schizophrenia.

Treatment

1. *Behaviour therapy*, using thought stopping, response prevention, or flooding, is the treatment of choice.

2. *Drugs:* the tricyclic antidepressant clomipramine appears to have specific benefits in obsessive-compulsive neurosis. It works best if depressed mood is also present. Other antidepressants, MAOIs, or anxiolytics are helpful in some cases.

3. *Psychotherapy:* supportive psychotherapy, including reassurance that disturbing obsessional thoughts have no basis in reality, is helpful as an adjunct to other treatments. Psychodynamic psychotherapy has been tried in the belief that obsessive-compulsive symptoms stem from conflicts in childhood, but has no proven benefit and has the danger of worsening the symptoms by increasing anxiety.

4. *Leucotomy:* this is only used for severe intractable cases, but its success rate for these is 60% which is higher than that for any other treatment.

Prognosis

The course often fluctuates, symptoms getting worse if the patient suffers a depressive mood swing or environmental stress. Mild cases may recover completely, but severe ones seldom do. About 5% of patients develop schizophrenia.

HYSTERIA (Merskey, 1979)

Definition

WHO definition: 'Mental disorders in which motives, of which the patient seems unaware, produce either a restriction of the field of consciousness or disturbance of motor or sensory function which may seem to have psychological advantage or symbolic value' (World Health Organization, 1978).

Hysteria is diagnosed when a symptom, physical or mental, arises in the absence of any other disease, the patient acquires some gain from the symptom, and is inappropriately unconcerned about it (*'la belle indifference'*). It has been argued that hysteria does not exist as a discrete entity, and that 'hysterical' symptoms are always a manifestation of another undiagnosed condition, but the concept has continued to be clinically useful (Lewis, 1975).

Prevalence

No figures are available. Hysteria is rarer in Britain today than formerly.

Epidemiology and Aetiology

1. *Age:* most common in early adult life.

2. *Sex:* more common in women.

3. *Cultural background:* hysteria is more common in underdeveloped countries, and in those of below average education in developed countries. This may be because it is unacceptable to express psychological complaints directly in these social groups.

4. *Premorbid personality:* often of 'hysterical' type (Chapter 6), with neurotic characteristics and tendency to extraversion.

5. *Organic brain disease* is sometimes present.

6. *Psychological stress* often precipitates episodes. Freud believed that hysteria resulted from repression of an anxiety-provoking trauma, followed by dissociation, and expression of the anxiety in the form of a symptom which by its nature had a symbolic relationship with the original trauma. This process dissipated the anxiety, resulting in indifference towards the symptom.

7. *Genetic factors* are insignificant, which is unusual in psychiatric syndromes, and supports the theory that hysteria is not a separate entity.

Clinical Features

A wide variety of symptoms may occur, and the type displayed may depend on the patient's medical knowledge. Mental symptoms ('dissociation symptoms') include amnesia, fugues, trances, twilight states, multiple personality and pseudodementia. Physical symptoms ('conversion symptoms') are usually neurological, and include paralyses, fits, pain, anaesthesia, and blindness. Other physical symptoms include vomiting, hyperventilation, and pseudocyesis. Epidemics of the same hysterical symptom may occur, e.g. vomiting among children in a school, fainting in members of a crowd.

Gains which may result from the hysterical symptom include escape from unwelcome obligations, e.g. the 'shell-shocked' soldier in the First World War rendered unable to fight by a hysterical paralysis; escape from the consequences of a crime, e.g. amnesia in one accused of murder; or the acquisition of sympathy and attention for a lonely, unhappy person.

Briquet's syndrome (St. Louis hysteria) is the development of 25 or more somatic hysterical symptoms in a young women (Editorial, 1977). Hysterical mechanisms may underlie some other syndromes described in psychiatry: Munchausen's syndrome (Chapter 16), Ganser syndrome (Chapter 16), and 'compensation neurosis' (Chapter 8).

Differential Diagnosis

1. *Organic disease*, especially neurological.

2. *Psychiatric illness:* hysterical symptoms may be secondary to depression, schizophrenia, or dementia.

3. *Malingering:* this differs from hysteria in that symptoms are deliberately feigned, rather than produced by unconscious mechanisms. Differentiation between hysteria and malingering may be impossible.

Treatment

Treatment is aimed at revealing the patient's repressed problems. This may be attempted by exploratory psychotherapy, if necessary with the aid of drugs (abreaction) or hypnosis. Physical examination and appropriate investigations are necessary to rule out organic disease, but should not be unduly extensive if there are positive grounds for thinking that the symptom is hysterical.

Prognosis

About 50% of acute episodes recover but recurrences, with the same symptom or others, are frequent. In a long-term follow-up study (Slater, 1965) it was found that about a third of patients originally diagnosed as hysterical turned out to have organic neurological disease or a psychotic illness.

References

Beech, H. R. (Ed.). (1974). *Obsessional States*. Methuen, London.
Editorial (1977). Briquet's syndrome or hysteria? *Lancet* i, 1138–1139.
Lewis, A. (1975). The survival of hysteria. *Psychol. Med.* **5**, 9–12.
Marks, I. M. (1969). *Fears and phobias*. Heinemann, London.
Marks, I. M., and Lader, M. (1973). Anxiety states (anxiety neurosis): a review. *J. Nerv. Ment. Dis.* **156**, 3–18.
Merskey, H. (1979). *The Analysis of Hysteria*. Baillière Tindall, London.
Murray, R. M. and Reveley, A. (1981). The genetic contribution to the neuroses. *Br. J. Hosp. Med.* **25**, 185–190.
Slater, E. (1965). Diagnosis of 'hysteria'. *Br. Med. J.* **1**, 1395–1399.
Taylor, J. A. (1953). A personality scale of manifest anxiety. *J. Abnorm. Psychol.* **48**, 285–290.
World Health Organization (1978). *Mental Disorders: Glossary and Guide to their Classification in Accordance with the Ninth Revision of the International Classification of Diseases*. WHO, Geneva.

CHAPTER 6

Personality Disorders

Definition

An extreme and persistent variation from the normal range of one or more personality attributes, resulting in suffering for the subject or for others.

There is no clear-cut dividing line between the normal and disordered personality, less severe abnormalities only being apparent under stress, and not all cases of personality disorder fit neatly into any of the types described below.

Before diagnosing personality disorder, it is essential to have evidence that the abnormalities have been present throughout the patient's adult life, and do not result from physical disease of the brain.

Classification

The eight types of abnormal personality described in ICD-9 (World Health Organization, 1978) are:

1. *Paranoid:* suspicious, prone to self-reference and to the development of overvalued ideas. Some subjects are sensitive and vulnerable, others aggressive about their rights.

2. *Affective:* consistent anomalies of mood are present, whether depression, cheerfulness (hyperthymic personality), or alternating phases of each (cyclothymic personality).

3. *Schizoid:* shy, reserved, introspective, often eccentric.

4. *Explosive:* subjects are usually pleasant and conformist but have sudden outbursts of extreme anger or impulsive behaviour.

5. *Anancastic (obsessive–compulsive):* insecure, cautious, stubborn, conscientious, perfectionist, with high ethical standards.

6. *Hysterical:* subjects with shallow and labile emotions, dependent on others but unreliable in relationships, and prone to dramatize situations.

7. *Asthenic:* lacking the energy and resilience to cope with even the everyday demands of life, and sometimes excessively dependent on others.

8. *Antisocial (sociopathic, psychopathic):* subjects show repeated anti-social behaviour, not modified by experience or punishment. They may be cold, callous, aggressive, and irresponsible. This type will be discussed in more detail below, since it is the one which most often comes to psychiatric attention, and the only one for which the Mental Health Act 1959 permits compulsory treatment.

The term 'psychopathy' may be used for all personality disorders, or only the antisocial type.

Relationship with Psychiatric Illness

Personality disorders appear to predispose to psychiatric illness, and the illness is often of a corresponding type, e.g. schizophrenia tends to develop in schizoid personalities, bipolar affective disorder in cyclothymic personalities, hysterical neurosis in hysterical personalities, obsessional neurosis in anancastic personalities. The relationship is difficult to investigate as it is hard to assess patients' personalities while they are ill, and retrospective assessments are unreliable.

Although personality disorder and psychiatric illness are considered to be separate phenomena, the differentiation between them may be impossible without long-term observation and independent accounts of the patient's usual previous behaviour.

Patients with personality disorders are liable to come to psychiatric attention even if there is no superimposed psychiatric illness, as they often have difficulties in adjustment to life, and may consequently develop emotional problems or abuse drugs and alcohol.

Treatment

Personality disorders, by definition, involve long-standing characteristics which are not amenable to radical change. However, it may be possible to modify undesirable traits and their ill-effects by psycho-therapy aiming to give the subject greater insight and improved behaviour patterns.

ANTISOCIAL PERSONALITY DISORDER

The Mental Health Act 1959 (using the term 'psychopathy') gives this definition:

'A persistent disorder or disability of mind (whether or not including subnormality of intelligence) which results in abnormally aggressive or seriously irresponsible conduct on the part of the patient, and requires or is susceptible to medical treatment.'

The history of the concept is described by Lewis (1974).

Aetiology

1. *Genetic predisposition* is suggested by adoption studies.

2. *Mild brain damage*, including temporal lobe epilepsy or a history of brain damage in early life, is present in a few cases. About 50% have an immature EEG.

3. *A disturbed upbringing* is common, suggesting that the condition may partly result from lack of guidance about acceptable behaviour in child-hood.

4. *Personality studies* show that sociopaths are highly extraverted and therefore resistant to conditioning.

5. *The XYY sex chromosome* constitution is more common in sociopaths in secure hospitals than in the general population. However, most sociopaths have normal chromosomes, and the XYY constitution is not always associated with sociopathic traits.

Clinical Features

Sociopaths consistently behave in a way which is unacceptable in their culture (the majority of prison inmates have sociopathic traits), but seem unable to improve their behaviour. They seek immediate pleasures without considering the long-term consequences, and are unable to make lasting relationships with others although they are often skilled in casual contacts.

Inadequate, aggressive, and creative types were described by Henderson (1939).

Males predominate, and usually present in early adult life.

Differential Diagnosis

1. *Psychiatric illness*, e.g. hypomania.

2. *Organic conditions*, e.g. frontal lobe lesions, drug-induced states.

Treatment

Section 26 of the Mental Health Act 1959 provides for compulsory admission of sociopaths under the age of 21, and their detention until the age of 25, for treatment. This has been criticized, since there is no evidence that psychiatric treatment is effective at any age.

Group psychotherapy in a therapeutic community setting with other sociopaths in institutions like the Henderson Hospital or Grendon Underwood Prison is beneficial in about 40% of cases.

Individual psychotherapy is seldom successful as patients may be manipulative, or unreliable in attendance.

Drugs seldom help and are often abused.

Patients with a temporal lobe abnormality may benefit from anti-convulsants, or excision of the area.

Prognosis

Overtly antisocial conduct usually diminishes with age, but difficulties with adjustment often remain a lifelong problem. About 5% of sociopaths die by suicide. The aggressive ones have the worst prognosis.

Further Reading

A classical text on abnormal personalities is that by Schneider (1950). Antisocial personality disorder is discussed in books by Cleckley (1976) and Craft (1966), and a paper by Whiteley (1970).

References

Cleckley, H. (1976). *The Mask of Sanity: An Attempt to Clarify some Issues about the So-Called Psychopathic Personality*. C. V. Mosby Company, St. Louis.

Craft, M. (1966). *Psychopathic Disorders*. Pergamon, Oxford.

Henderson, D. (1939). *Psychopathic States*. W. W. Norton, New York.

Lewis, A. (1974). Psychopathic personality: a most elusive category. *Psychol. Med.*, **4**, 133–140.

Schneider, K. (1950). *Psychopathic Personalities*. Trans. M. W. Hamilton, 1958. Cassell, London.

Whiteley, J. S. (1970). The psychopath and his treatment. *Br. J. Hosp. Med.*, **3**, 263–270.

World Health Organization (1978). *Mental Disorders: Glossary and Guide to their Classification in Accordance with the Ninth Revision of the International Classification of Diseases*. WHO, Geneva.

CHAPTER 7

Organic Psychiatry I

ORGANIC BRAIN SYNDROMES

Organic brain syndromes (organic psychoses) are conditions in which mental dysfunction is secondary to organic pathology.

Causes of Organic Brain Syndromes

1. *Cerebral conditions:*
   (a) Degenerative, e.g. senile dementia, presenile dementias, Parkinson's disease.
   (b) Space-occupying lesions, e.g. tumour, subdural haematoma.
   (c) Infections, e.g. encephalitis, meningitis, syphilis.
   (d) Head injury.
   (e) Epilepsy.
   (f) Vascular, e.g. arteriosclerosis, stroke, hypertensive encephalopathy, collagen diseases.
   (g) Miscellaneous, e.g. multiple sclerosis, normal pressure hydrocephalus, Wilson's disease.

2. *Systemic conditions:*
   (a) Infections, e.g. septicaemia, pneumonia.
   (b) Metabolic disturbances, e.g. renal or hepatic failure, electrolyte imbalance, remote effects of carcinoma, porphyria.
   (c) Endocrine disorders.
   (d) Poisons, e.g. alcohol and drug intoxication or withdrawal, heavy metals.
   (e) Cardiac or respiratory conditions causing cerebral anoxia.
   (f) Vitamin B deficiency.

Clinical Features of Organic Brain Syndromes

Organic cerebral disorders usually present with clouding of consciousness or cognitive impairment, which may be accompanied by neurological symptoms or signs. The clinical picture is called delirium in acute cases, and dementia in chronic ones; these syndromes are described below.

Less often, organic cases present with neurotic or psychotic symptoms resembling those found in functional disorders. Such cases may have atypical features suggesting an organic cause: fluctuation of the symptoms, visual hallucinations, vague or transient paranoid delusions, or first onset of neurotic symptoms in middle or old age. The opposite diagnostic difficulty may arise because some patients with acute functional psychoses also have slight clouding of consciousness and cognitive impairment. The investigation of organic cases is described in Chapter 2.

DELIRIUM

Delirium (acute brain syndrome, dysmnesic syndrome, toxic confusional state) is clouding of consciousness accompanied by abnormalities of perception, thought and mood, from an organic cause. The alcohol withdrawal syndrome (delirium tremens) is a common example.

The patient is confused and disorientated, restless and overactive, may have illusions, hallucinations of visual, auditory or tactile type, and changeable paranoid delusions. The severity fluctuates and is usually worse at night.

General management consists of intensive nursing care, attention to fluid and electrolyte balance, and sedation, for which phenothiazines are suitable. Confusion may be reduced by providing a well-lit single room with as few different nurses as possible. The underlying cause should be identified and treated.

Outcome depends on the cause and may be complete recovery, partial recovery with residual dementia, or death.

DEMENTIA

Dementia (chronic brain syndrome) is an acquired impairment of intellect and memory, often accompanied by changes in personality, mood, and behaviour, from an organic cause. It is chronic, and usually progressive and irreversible.

The 'primary dementias' include senile dementia and the presenile dementias which comprise Alzheimer's disease, Pick's disease, Huntington's chorea and Jakob–Creutzfeld disease. Dementia can also occur secondary to any of the conditions listed above as causes of organic brain syndromes. Senile dementia and arteriosclerotic dementia are the commonest causes. A general account of dementia is given first, and followed by a description of these individual types.

Clinical features: onset is usually gradual, unless the dementia is the sequel of a delirious illness. Memory loss is usually the first symptom; it involves recent rather than remote memories, and results in disorientation. Other intellectual functions also deteriorate. Affective changes are common, and may consist either of lability of mood, or a sustained depression or euphoria. Exaggeration of previous personality traits, and a coarsening of personality accompanied by socially unacceptable behaviour, may occur. Insight is usually absent, except in the early stages.

Diagnosis (Roth and Myers, 1969): diagnosis is usually obvious from the history and simple tests of cognitive function, but may be confirmed by formal psychological tests of intelligence and memory. Formal tests are more useful in monitoring the course of the condition than in diagnosis.

Investigation of cause: all cases require a full history and physical examination, and investigations to exclude treatable causes: blood count and ESR, urea and electrolytes, liver function tests, thyroid function tests, B_{12} and folate, calcium and phosphate, serological tests for syphilis, chest and skull X-ray. More extensive investigations may be required if these tests do not reveal the cause. These include an EEG, brain scan, and brain biopsy. They are only indicated if their results would alter treatment, and seldom justified in patients who are severely demented or very old.

Differential diagnosis: depression is the main condition with which dementia may be confused in the elderly. Depression and dementia can usually be distinguished by the history, mental state, and psychological testing, but in some patients the two coexist. In doubtful cases a trial of antidepressant treatment may be required to confirm the diagnosis.

Management: the underlying cause should be corrected if possible, but the majority of cases do not have a treatable cause. The aim of treatment is to keep patients functioning at their best possible level by maintenance of good physical health and provision of a suitable environment. Inpatient facilities are not adequate to cope with all the demented people in the country, but in any case it is thought best for patients to remain in their homes with help from community services (Chapter 17), as hospital admission often causes them to become distressed and even more confused. The burden on relatives can be lessened by arranging short 'holiday' admissions every few months, and making prompt emergency admission available in the event of intercurrent illness or a social crisis. When patients deteriorate so much that their families cannot care for them, permanent hospital care is necessary.

Affective or paranoid symptoms in demented patients should be treated with appropriate drugs. ECT is contraindicated in theory because it could exacerbate the dementia, but in practice may be beneficial when a demented patient is severely depressed.

Prognosis: in the few patients with a treatable cause, e.g. hypo-thyroidism, progression of the dementia can be arrested and there may even be partial recovery, but most cases gradually deteriorate. Acute confusional episodes due to other pathology, e.g. chest or urinary infection, small strokes, faecal impaction, or inappropriate medication, may occur and leave permanent residual damage.

Senile Dementia

Senile dementia is the commonest form of dementia. By definition, it only occurs after age 65, and it affects 5% of people over this age, becoming more frequent as age increases. It is nearly twice as common in women as in men. There is genetic predisposition to its development. The pathology represents an extreme form of the normal changes of old age. All organs of the body shrink. Shrinkage of the brain results in enlargement of the ventricles and sulci. Neurones are decreased both in number and size, and astrocytes proliferate. Senile plaques, which have argyrophylic cores containing an amyloid-like substance, form in the grey matter. Nerve fibres form tangles called Alzheimer's neurofibrillary degeneration. Post-mortem brain studies have shown a deficiency of the enzyme choline acetyltransferase, which is concerned in the synthesis of acetylcholine, and it is believed that defective cholinergic transmission may be important in causing the symptoms. Cerebral blood flow and oxygen consumption are reduced. The EEG usually shows theta or delta waves, and alpha rhythm is slow or absent.

Onset is gradual, over a year or more. Loss of recent memory is usually the first symptom, and is followed by deterioration in other intellectual functions, emotional lability or depression, and personality change. Delusions and hallucinations occur in advanced cases. Insight is usually absent, and the patient comes to medical attention because relatives or neighbours notice failing memory, confusion, or inability to cope with basic self-care.

There is no specific treatment although trials of choline are currently in progress. Most patients die from pneumonia about five years after the onset of their dementia.

Arteriosclerotic Dementia

Arteriosclerotic or 'multi-infarct' dementia is almost as common as senile dementia. The two conditions are pathologically quite different, but may coexist by chance. Arteriosclerotic dementia usually starts in the 60s, but sometimes much earlier. Men are affected slightly more often than women.

The pathology is focal infarction of the brain due to haemorrhage, thrombosis, or embolism associated with cerebral arteriosclerosis. Most patients have hypertension, focal neurological signs, and evidence of arteriosclerosis in other organs.

Loss of memory, intellectual deterioration, and affective changes occur, but insight and personality are retained better than in senile dementia. Deterioration is stepwise rather than gradual, as repeated small strokes or episodes of hypertensive encephalopathy take place and leave residual damage.

Some cases might be prevented by control of hypertension in its early stages, and attention to potential sources of cerebral emboli. There is no established treatment for the condition once developed; vasodilator drugs have been tried with little success. The average survival time is about five years, and the usual causes of death are ischaemic heart disease and stroke.

Alzheimer's Disease

Alzheimer's disease is the commonest of the primary presenile dementias. Onset is between the ages of 40 and 60, and women are affected at least twice as often as men. Most cases arise sporadically but others are inherited, either in polygenic fashion or by a dominant gene. There is no genetic link with senile dementia, although the pathology of both conditions is apparently the same.

Memory disturbance is the first symptom and develops gradually over two or three years. There is then a rapid intellectual deterioration with symptoms of parietal lobe dysfunction (dysphasia, apraxia, agnosia, acalculia), accompanied by extrapyramidal signs. Terminal cases have severe dementia and marked neurological abnormalities. The EEG is always abnormal, with theta and delta waves and reduced alpha rhythm. Death occurs two to five years after the onset.

Pick's Disease

Pick's disease is rarer than Alzheimer's disease. Onset is between the ages of 50 and 60, and women are affected twice as often as men. A dominant gene is probably the cause.

Cerebral atrophy occurs, with loss of neurones and gliosis, and is most marked in the frontal and temporal lobes.

Symptoms of frontal lobe damage (disinhibited behaviour, and reduction of drive, without insight) occur first and are followed by impairment of memory and intellect. Dysphasia, apraxia, agnosia, and extrapyramidal symptoms are sometimes present. The EEG may show non-specific abnormalities or may be normal. Death occurs two to ten years after the onset.

Jakob–Creutzfeld Disease (Creutzfeld–Jakob Disease)

Jakob–Creutzfeld disease is a rare form of presenile dementia. Onset may be at any age, but most often between the ages of 30 and 50. Men and women are affected equally.

The condition does not run in families. A viral cause is suspected because some cases have developed following surgery with infected instruments, and it can be experimentally transmitted to monkeys.

Dementia and diverse neurological abnormalities both develop rapidly, and death occurs within two years. Amantadine has been tried in treatment with some success.

Huntington's Chorea (Office of Health Economics, 1980)

Huntington's chorea is a rare form of inherited presenile dementia which is important because of its genetic aspects. It affects 5 per 100,000 of the population, but there is regional variation. Onset may be at any age, but most often between 35 and 45. Men and women are affected equally. An autosomal dominant gene with complete penetrance is the cause. 50% of the children of an affected parent will develop the condition, and because of the late age of onset, many patients have already had children by the time the disease begins. Occasional cases have no family history; these may be spontaneous mutations or be illegitimate.

There is generalized atrophy of the brain, most severe in the frontal lobes, caudate nuclei, and putamen. Deficiency of the neurotransmitter GABA and excess of dopamine have both been demonstrated at post-mortem.

Choreiform movements and dementia are the most characteristic symptoms but there may be any type of psychiatric abnormality. There is great variation in the order in which symptoms develop, and in the course of the disease, but the average survival is about 15 years. The chorea can be treated with phenothiazines or tetrabenazine, and any psychiatric symptoms present should be treated with appropriate drugs.

If there was a reliable test to identify carriers of the gene, they could be advised not to have children and new cases therefore prevented. At present there is no such test; some early cases show characteristic eye movements, a low voltage EEG, and develop choreiform movements if given L-dopa, but these findings are not diagnostic.

More organic conditions which may cause delirium, dementia, or other psychiatric symptoms are described in Chapter 8; the effects of alcohol in Chapter 9, and of drug abuse in Chapter 10.

Further Reading

A comprehensive book on organic psychiatry is that by Lishman (1978).

References

Lishman, W. A. (1978). *Organic Psychiatry*. Blackwell Scientific Publications, Oxford.

Office of Health Economics (1980). *Huntington's Chorea*. OHE, London.

Roth, M., and Myers, D. (1969). The diagnosis of dementia. *Br. J. Hosp. Med.*, **2**, 705–717.

CHAPTER 8

Organic Psychiatry II

INTERACTIONS BETWEEN PSYCHIATRIC AND PHYSICAL ILLNESS

Twenty-five to fifty per cent of medical inpatients have psychiatric symptoms, and a similar proportion of psychiatric patients have physical ones (Maguire and Granville-Grossman, 1968; Maguire *et al.*, 1974). Reasons for the association include:

1. *Organic brain syndromes* (Chapter 7): organic pathology directly affects cerebral function.

2. *Maladaptive psychological reactions to physical illness* (Lloyd, 1977): the illness, and any changes in social circumstances which result from it, may act as 'life events', precipitating depression or other psychiatric symptoms. Loss of a body part, e.g. amputation of a limb (Parkes, 1975) seems especially prone to cause depression. Depression or anxiety may delay physical recovery. In some patients hysterical mechanisms cause symptoms to persist after their physical basis has recovered, enabling them to gain attention or compensation or avoid responsibility.

3. *'Psychosomatic' disease:* psychological stress is believed to be a causative factor in some physical diseases. Seven supposedly psychosomatic diseases were described in the 1930s: rheumatoid arthritis, ulcerative colitis, bronchial asthma, essential hypertension, neurodermatitis, thyrotoxicosis, and peptic ulcer. The suggested mechanism is that in people with a characteristic personality structure and vulnerability of a certain physical system, psychological stress leads to autonomic, endocrine, or immunological changes which cause disease. There are methodological problems in demonstrating that psychosomatic mechanisms exist, but many studies suggest that they do, e.g. ischaemic heart disease appears to be more common in men of 'Type A' personality (Editorial, 1980), an excess of life events has been reported

prior to myocardial infarction (Connolly, 1976), and mortality from cardiovascular conditions is increased in widowers after bereavement (Parkes *et al.*, 1969).

4. *Psychiatric conditions may present with physical complaints*, e.g. the physical symptoms of anxiety, hypochondriacal preoccupations or delusions in depressive illness, hysterical conversion symptoms, and the Munchausen syndrome. Physical damage may result from drug or alcohol abuse, deliberate self-harm, or self-neglect.

5. *Medical treatment* may have psychological side-effects, e.g. hypotensive drugs can cause depression.

PSYCHIATRIC ASPECTS OF SOME NEUROLOGICAL AND MEDICAL CONDITIONS

Epilepsy (Scott, 1978)

Epilepsy affects 5 per 1000 of the population. Psychiatric disturbance is present in about 30% of patients with epilepsy, and about 50% of those with temporal lobe epilepsy. Reasons for the high prevalence include:

1. The brain lesion responsible for the epilepsy may also cause psychiatric symptoms.
2. Brain damage from anoxia may result from frequent fits.
3. Abnormal electrophysiological activity is present between fits in some patients and impairs mental functioning.
4. Anticonvulsant drugs can impair intellectual function directly, or indirectly by disturbing folic acid or calcium metabolism.
5. Psychosocial consequences of epilepsy; epileptics are often treated differently, whether stigmatized or overprotected, and denied full social and educational opportunities. Personality problems and neurotic symptoms may result.

Cognitive function: uncomplicated epilepsy does not have an association with low intelligence, but in a minority of patients one or more of the factors listed above impedes intellectual development, or causes dementia in later life.

Personality: about 50% of patients with temporal lobe epilepsy have an abnormal personality. Aggressive outbursts are the most frequent characteristic, and impulsiveness, suspiciousness, sensitivity, and moodiness are other features. These traits may be due to structural or functional abnormalities of the limbic system, and often improve following excision of a localized focus. A typical 'epileptic personality' used to be described among institutionalized patients, characterized by untrustworthiness, subservience, aggressiveness, paranoid traits, and religiosity, but it is no longer believed that this is a valid entity.

Neuroses: neurotic symptoms are more frequent among epileptics than in the general population. Depression and irritability may be present for a few days before a fit.

Psychoses (Flor-Henry, 1969; Slater *et al.*, 1963)
1. Transient episodes with hallucinations, usually visual or auditory, and delusions, usually paranoid, accompanied by clouding of consciousness, may occur in association with fits. The EEG may show 'forced normalization' during these attacks.
2. Schizophrenia develops with greater than expected frequency in patients with temporal lobe epilepsy of the dominant hemisphere. Paranoid schizophrenia is the commonest type.
3. Affective disorders, especially depression, also occur with greater than expected frequency and are associated with temporal lobe epilepsy of the non-dominant hemisphere.

The conventional treatments for psychotic symptoms can safely be used in epilepsy; although ECT, phenothiazines, and tricyclics could theoretically increase fit frequency, in practice this is rare.

Suicide: suicide is about five times more common in epileptics than in the general population.

Sexual disorders: temporal lobe epilepsy is often associated with hyposexuality. Sexually deviant behaviour is occasionally associated with temporal lobe seizures or localized brain lesions.

Crime: criminal behaviour is slightly more common among epileptics than in the general population, and epileptics are over-represented in prison. Motiveless violent crimes may be committed in the post-ictal state, but this is very rare.

Differential diagnosis of epilepsy: sometimes epilepsy is impossible to diagnose with confidence especially if there are psychomotor seizures without convulsions. Psychiatric conditions in the differential diagnosis are the phobic anxiety depersonalization syndrome, schizophrenia, hysteria, drug or alcohol intoxication, explosive personality disorder, and simulation. Physical conditions which may be misdiagnosed as epilepsy include syncope, cardiac arrhythmias, hypoglycaemic attacks, transient ischaemic attacks, and migraine.

Head Injury (Lishman, 1973)

Head injuries, mostly resulting from road traffic accidents, cause at least 100,000 hospital admissions per year in the UK. The effects of head injury depend on the site, size, and extent of the brain damage, and on the patient's reaction as determined by age, premorbid personality, the circumstances of the accident, and its social consequences.

Organic changes: epilepsy, usually temporal lobe epilepsy, develops after 5% of closed head injuries, and after 30–50% of penetrating injuries, but may not start for several years afterwards. It is commoner if fits occurred immediately following the injury, and if post-traumatic amnesia was longer than 24 hours. Treatment is with anticonvulsants, or by excision of the epileptogenic focus.

Cognitive defects occur after 2–3% of head injuries. They are more common with severe injuries, and if post-traumatic amnesia was longer than 24 hours, and are often associated with neurological defects. Closed injuries lead to a global impairment of cognitive functions whereas open injuries cause more circumscribed impairment. Most cases improve over the following two years. Cognitive defects may be exaggerated by psychiatric symptoms, or by physical complications such as subdural haematoma.

Personality change: up to 20% of patients develop frontal lobe symptoms of apathy, disinhibition and mild euphoria. Damage to the amygdala may cause aggressive behaviour.

Psychoses develop in about 8% of patients. Schizophrenic symptoms tend to be associated with temporal lobe injuries. Paranoid states and depressive illness may occur; mania is rare. Antipsychotic drugs are usually effective, and ECT can be used if they fail.

Neurotic symptoms such as anxiety, depression, irritability, obsessive-compulsive symptoms, and hysterical conversion symptoms develop in up to 20% of patients. They may be helped by psychotherapy. The post-traumatic syndrome, or 'compensation neurosis' (Miller, 1961) comprises headache, dizziness, fatigue, irritability, and poor concentration. It is thought to be psychogenic, since it is unrelated to severity of injury or to organic impairments, but is commoner when compensation is pending and often recovers following settlement of compensation claims.

Social consequences of head injury are often adverse because working ability is impaired, and changes in personality and behaviour damage close relationships.

Suicide accounts for 14% of deaths in those who survive head injury.

Either improvement or deterioration may continue for years after a head injury, so that serial assessments are required. Repeated EEGs may help to tell when the patient's condition has become stable.

Chronic progressive traumatic encephalopathy (the 'punch-drunk' syndrome) affects boxers who get repeated minor head injuries. Cerebellar, extrapyramidal, and pyramidal signs are present and there is cognitive impairment. Cerebral atrophy occurs, and perforation of the septum pellucidum is a common finding.

Cerebral Tumours

Most patients with cerebral tumours have psychiatric symptoms, which may begin before there are any neurological abnormalities. Three per cent of psychiatric inpatients had an unsuspected tumour discovered at post-mortem in one series. The type of psychiatric symptom has limited value in localizing the tumour, as symptoms result from effects of intracranial pressure and displacement at other sites in the brain. Impaired consciousness, often fluctuating, is the commonest change. Mild dementia, including focal cognitive defects, is also frequent. Personality change, mood change, delusions, hallucinations, and neurotic symptoms may occur.

Parkinson's Disease (Mindham, 1974)

Cognitive impairment is present in 20–40% of patients. It is more common in arteriosclerotic Parkinsonism than in the idiopathic type, because of arteriosclerotic changes elsewhere in the brain.

Depression is present in 50–70% of patients. It appears to be part of the disease process itself, as distinct from the reactive depression which may occur in any chronic disease, and dopamine deficiency could be the cause.

Multiple Sclerosis (Surridge, 1969)

About 60% of patients have cognitive impairment; 50% have mood change. Depression is commoner in the early stages of the illness, and is usually of reactive type. Euphoria is commoner in the later stages of the illness and has an association with intellectual impairment.

Multiple sclerosis may be misdiagnosed as hysteria, because of the fluctuating symptoms and paucity of objective neurological signs in the initial stages.

Normal Pressure Hydrocephalus (Rice and Gendelman, 1973)

An obstruction in the subarachnoid space preventing CSF circulation, with normal intraventricular pressure, is present in this condition. Some cases result from a block in the basal cisterns due to local pathology. Brain scan shows very large ventricles, with no air surrounding the hemispheres.

Memory impairment and psychomotor retardation are the main psychiatric symptoms, and are accompanied by an unsteady gait and incontinence of urine. Severe dementia may develop.

Insertion of a ventriculocaval shunt may produce a great improvement.

Neurosyphilis

Meningovascular syphilis may cause headache, lethargy, malaise, mild intellectual impairment, and emotional lability. GPI may present with personality changes of frontal lobe type; cognitive impairment; or mood change, either euphoria with grandiose ideas or delusions, or depression. Less often there are schizophrenic symptoms, paranoid delusions, or an acute organic brain syndrome.

Neurological examination often shows cranial nerve palsies in meningovascular syphilis, and pupillary abnormalities, tremor, dysarthria or other signs in GPI. Serological tests (WR, VDRL, RPCF, TPI, FTA) may be negative on blood but are always positive on CSF. CSF also shows a lymphocytosis, raised protein, and a paretic Lange colloidal gold curve.

Treatment with penicillin may produce an improvement if given in the early stages.

Encephalitis

Encephalitis may be caused by viral infection of the brain itself, or follow a systemic viral illness (e.g. influenza, measles) probably due to an autoimmune process.

The presentation is usually with headache and fever, which may be accompanied by any psychiatric abnormality. Raised intracranial pressure and neurological signs are usually present, but subacute cases may have psychiatric symptoms without neurological abnormality. Permanent psychiatric sequelae may remain and include dementia, personality change with disinhibition and overactivity (especially in children), and obsessive–compulsive symptoms.

Encephalitis lethargica has been extensively studied although it became a rare disease after the epidemics of 1918–20. Its sequelae included Parkinsonism, oculogyric crises, obsessive–compulsive symptoms, sleepiness by day, and psychoses.

The depressive symptoms which may be present for several months after infectious mononucleosis and infectious hepatitis may be due to a similar process.

Endocrine Conditions (Gibbons, 1974)

Hypothyroidism: psychiatric symptoms are always present, and may be the most prominent ones. Slowing of mental processes, poor memory, and depressed mood are usual, so that the condition is easily mis-diagnosed as dementia or depressive illness. An acute psychiatric episode occasionally occurs ('myxoedema madness') with features of delirium or of an acute psychosis with paranoid delusions.

Hyperthyroidism: psychiatric symptoms are always present, usually those of an anxiety state. Occasional cases present with symptoms of mania, agitated depression, schizophrenia, or paranoid delusions. A thyrotoxic crisis may present with delirium.

Cushing's syndrome: both Cushing's syndrome and steroid therapy produce mood changes of depression, euphoria, or emotional lability in about 80% of patients. Cushing's syndrome usually causes depression, whereas euphoria is more common in patients on steroid therapy. Less often acute psychotic symptoms occur.

Addison's disease: psychiatric symptoms are always present, and include apathy, depression, anxiety, and memory impairment. Addisonian crisis can cause delirium because of electrolyte imbalance.

Hypopituitarism: psychiatric symptoms are usually present and include apathy, depression, and memory impairment. Hypopituitarism occurring after childbirth may be misdiagnosed as post-partum depression.

Hypoglycaemia: the episodic alterations of consciousness and dis-inhibited behaviour in hypoglycaemic attacks may stimulate psychiatric illness or epilepsy. Prolonged hypoglycaemia can cause brain damage and dementia.

Diabetes: hyperglycaemia may cause delirium. Diabetics may develop cerebral arteriosclerosis with resultant dementia or psychiatric symptoms. Diabetic neuropathy can cause impotence, which may be misdiagnosed as psychogenic.

Hyperparathyroidism: about 60% of patients have psychiatric symptoms, usually depression and apathy, occasionally without any physical complaints. Organic brain syndromes may occur.

Hypoparathyroidism: about 50% of patients have psychiatric symptoms, including intellectual impairment, anxiety, and depression.

Psychiatric symptoms secondary to endocrine disorders should respond to treatment of the underlying condition unless they are very long-standing, in which case they need treatment on their own merits and even then may not disappear completely.

Cancer

The following mechanisms may lead to psychiatric symptoms in cancer patients.

1. *Cerebral metastases:* multiple deposits, single deposits, or diffuse infiltration of the brain and meninges by tumour cells, may give rise to neuropsychiatric symptoms.

2. *'Remote effects'* including encephalopathy, myelopathy, neuropathy, and myopathy may develop in the absence of cerebral metastases,

especially in patients with lung cancer. The course of such syndromes is unrelated to that of the tumour. They may result from virus infection, immunological impairment, hormone secretion, or metabolic disturbance. Presentation may be with dementia, affective changes, or neurological signs.

3. *Knowledge of the diagnosis of cancer* may precipitate depression, anxiety or other psychiatric symptoms.

4. *Treatments* such as extensive surgery, radiotherapy, or cytotoxic drugs may cause depression.

5. *An association between depressive illness and cancer*, especially cancer of the pancreas, has been reported but remains unproven.

Liver Failure

Acute episodes of neuropsychiatric disturbance may be precipitated by a high protein intake, or other metabolic disturbance, in patients with liver disease. Clouded consciousness with visual hallucinations, memory impairment, and hypersomnia are accompanied by neurological abnormalities of which flapping tremor is most characteristic. The EEG shows theta waves and slowing of alpha rhythm, and EEG changes correlate with the severity of the condition.

Changes in between acute episodes include mood swings, and personality changes of frontal lobe type, but any psychiatric symptom may occur.

Porphyria

Porphyria is inherited as an autosomal dominant of incomplete penetrance, involves defects of haemoglobin metabolism, and has several varieties of which the Swedish and South African are most common. There are intermittent attacks of abdominal pain, neuropathy, and varied psychiatric symptoms. Attacks can be precipitated by drugs (barbiturates, sulphonamides, griseofulvin, oestrogens) and by pregnancy.

Wilson's Disease (Hepatolenticular Degeneration)

Wilson's disease is a famous but rare condition inherited as an autosomal recessive, and involves a deficiency of the copper-transporting substance caeruloplasmin. Copper is deposited in the basal ganglia, liver, kidney, and eye, causing choreoathetosis, dementia, schizophreniform symptoms, cirrhosis, aminoaciduria, and a Kayser–Fleischer ring.

Collagen Diseases

About 50% of patients with systemic lupus erythematosus or polyarteritis nodosa have psychiatric symptoms and the same is probably true in other collagen diseases. Organic brain syndromes, psychotic symptoms, and neurotic symptoms occur in that order of frequency. Episodes are often transient. The psychiatric manifestations are due to the disease process itself, usually to vasculitis of cerebral vessels, or to steroids used in treatment.

Deficiency Diseases

Vitamin B$_{12}$ deficiency (pernicious anaemia): depression, delirium, dementia, or paranoid states may occur, sometimes prior to any physical symptoms.

Folic acid deficiency: this is frequent among psychiatric patients, and may also result from anticonvulsant medication, but its exact significance is not known.

Nicotinic acid deficiency (pellagra): extreme mood changes, or delirium, may occur.

Further Reading

The list of conditions included in this chapter is not comprehensive; psychiatric symptoms can occur in association with almost any physical illness. A very detailed account is contained in the book on organic psychiatry by Lishman (1978).

References

Connolly, J. (1976). Life events before myocardial infarction. *J. Human Stress*, **2**, 3-17.
Editorial (1980). Type A behaviour and ischaemic heart disease. *Psychol. Med.*, **10**, 603-606.
Flor-Henry, P. (1969). Psychosis and temporal lobe epilepsy: a controlled investigation. *Epilepsia*, **10**, 363-395.

Gibbons, J. L. (1974). Editorial: Endocrinology and psychiatry. *Psychol. Med.*, **4**, 240–243.

Lishman, W. A. (1973). The psychiatric sequelae of head injury: a review. *Psychol. Med.*, **3**, 304–318.

Lishman, W. A. (1978). *Organic Psychiatry*. Blackwell Scientific Publications, Oxford.

Lloyd, G. G. (1977). Psychological reactions to physical illness. *Br. J. Hosp. Med.*, **18**, 352–358.

Maguire, G. P., and Granville-Grossman, K. L. (1968). Physical illness in psychiatric patients. *Br. J. Psychiatry*, **114**, 1365–1369.

Maguire, G. P., Julier, D. L., Hawton, K. E., and Bancroft, J. H. J. (1974). Psychiatric morbidity and referral on two general medical wards. *Br. Med. J.*, **1**, 268–270.

Miller, H. (1961). Accident neurosis. *Br. Med. J.*, **1**, 919–925 and 992–998.

Mindham, R. H. S. (1974). Psychiatric aspects of Parkinson's disease. *Br. J. Hosp. Med.*, **11**, 411–414.

Parkes, C. M. (1975). Psycho-social transitions: comparison between reactions to loss of a limb and loss of a spouse. *Br. J. Psychiatry*, **127**, 204–210.

Parkes, C. M., Benjamin, B., and Fitzgerald, R. G. (1969). Broken heart: a statistical study of increased mortality among widowers. *Br. Med. J.*, **1**, 740–743.

Rice, E., and Gendelman, S. (1973). Psychiatric aspects of normal pressure hydrocephalus. *JAMA*, **223**, 409–412.

Scott, D. F. (1978). Psychiatric aspects of epilepsy. *Br. J. Psychiatry*, **132**, 417–430.

Slater, E., Beard, A. W., and Clithero, E. (1963). The schizophrenia-like psychoses of epilepsy. *Br. J. Psychiatry*, **109**, 95–150.

Surridge, D. (1969). An investigation into some psychiatric aspects of multiple sclerosis. *Br. J. Psychiatry*, **115**, 749–764.

CHAPTER 9

Alcohol Abuse

Alcohol abuse is a major problem in Britain today and therefore considerable space is devoted to it here.

Definition of Alcoholism

There is no agreed demarcation between 'alcoholism' and heavy drinking. Alcoholism has been defined in terms of:

1. amount and frequency of drinking.
2. physical dependency on alcohol.
3. presence of alcohol-related disability, whether physical, mental, or social.

The WHO definition (1952): 'Alcoholics are those excessive drinkers whose dependence on alcohol has attained such a degree that they show a noticeable mental disturbance or an interference with their mental and bodily health, their interpersonal relations and their smooth economic and social functioning, or who show prodromal signs of such developments.'

Alcohol-related problems are likely to develop if daily alcohol consumption exceeds 4 pints of beer, or 4 doubles of spirits, or 1 bottle of wine (about 50 grams of alcohol).

Prevalence

Prevalence cannot be measured exactly because there is no agreed definition of alcoholism, and drinking is often concealed. Methods of estimating prevalence include:

1. community surveys.
2. hospital admissions for alcoholism.
3. mortality from cirrhosis.
4. convictions for drunkenness and drunken driving.
5. national per capita consumption of alcohol.

About 1% of the population of England and Wales have a serious drinking problem, and the percentage is increasing.

Epidemiology and Aetiology

1. *Sex:* formerly three times commoner in men, but becoming relatively more common in women.

2. *Age:* the majority present in middle age, but a growing proportion of cases are presenting in young adult life.

3. *Marital status:* 50% of those presenting for treatment are divorced or separated, usually as a result of their drinking.

4. *Social class:* classes I and V are over-represented.

5. *Occupation:* publicans, others in the alcohol trade, businessmen, seamen, journalists, and doctors are over-represented.

6. *Nationality:* France and Italy are the countries with the highest rates of alcohol-related problems. Britain is twelfth. Scotland and Ireland have higher rates than England. Jews and Arabs have very low rates. The national and occupational differences probably depend on the price and availability of alcohol, and culturally determined drinking norms.

7. *Genetics* (Shields, 1977): there is a 2–3-fold increase in alcoholism in the relatives of alcoholics, especially male ones; a higher concordance for alcoholism between monozygotic than dizygotic twins; and a high rate in children of alcoholic parents who were adopted into non-alcoholic homes in infancy. However, anyone can develop physical dependence on alcohol if they drink enough.

8. *Psychological factors:* stress is often the precipitant for heavy drinking, as alcohol is so effective as a temporary anxiolytic and euphoriant. Many alcoholics seem to have had premorbid personality disorders, but since alcohol abuse itself leads to personality changes, retrospective judgements are difficult to make. Psychiatric illness, most often depression, leads to the excess drinking in a few cases. Psychoanalytic theories explain alcoholisms in terms of oral dependency, latent homosexuality or self-destructive urges.

Alcoholism probably results from a mixture of individual predisposition, whether physical or psychological, and cultural factors.

Effects of Alcohol

Damage may result from the direct toxicity of ethanol, or from associated phenomena including vitamin B deficiency, hypoglycaemia, dehydration, overhydration, alcohol withdrawal, toxic congeners, and trauma sustained during intoxication.

Complications include liver damage, neurological and psychiatric syndromes, peptic ulcer, pancreatitis, gastritis, cardiomyopathy, myopathy, gout, vitamin deficiencies, and raised susceptibility to infections, including tuberculosis, and to malignancies. The mortality rate in alcoholics is three times higher than that of the general population.

Heavy drinking in pregnancy may cause abortion, stillbirth, or the 'fetal alcohol syndrome' comprising mental handicap, microcephaly, and various deformities.

Acute intoxication initially causes increased well-being, reduced inhibitions, and reduced efficiency (seldom recognized by the subject). Changes are obvious to an observer when blood alcohol is about 50 mg%. Heavier intoxication leads to emotional display of jocularity, sentimentality or aggression; intellectual impairment; ataxia and slurred speech from cerebellar effects; slow reaction time; vomiting; sometimes fits; and eventually coma, which occurs when blood alcohol is about 300 mg%. Coma may result from head injury, drug overdose, a recent fit, hypothermia, or hypoglycaemia, as well as from intoxication itself. Subsequent amnesia is usual.

Blood alcohol levels over 500 mg% may be fatal. Less severe intoxication may cause death through accidents or inhalation of vomit.

'Pathological intoxication' is abnormal behaviour following only modest alcohol intake, usually seen in brain-damaged people.

Liver damage includes acute hepatitis, fatty infiltration, and cirrhosis. Cirrhosis seldom develops until heavy drinking, of half a bottle of spirits or its equivalent daily, has continued for at least 5 years, although in women it may develop after a lower intake than this. Cirrhosis has a 5-year mortality rate of 50% in those who continue to drink, but is seldom fatal in those who become totally abstinent. A raised blood level of gamma glutamyltranspeptidase is a sensitive indicator of alcoholic liver damage which may assist diagnosis of a suspected case.

Delirium tremens seldom develops unless a patient has been drinking heavily for at least ten years. It can be precipitated by withdrawal of alcohol, by a heavy drinking bout, or by an operation or intercurrent illness. Patients appear severely ill, are confused, febrile, with visual or tactile hallucinations, and may have fits. Treatment is with a phenothiazine, chlormethiazole, or a benzodiazepine to counteract withdrawal symptoms and sedate the patient, correction of any fluid or electrolyte imbalance or hypoglycaemia, an anticonvulsant if required, and parenteral vitamins.

Wernicke's encephalopathy results from deficiency of vitamin B_1 (thiamine). Haemorrhages occur in the mammillary bodies, thalamus and hypothalamus. There is acute confusion with nystagmus, diplopia, ataxia, and peripheral neuritis. It may be fatal, unless treated with thiamine.

Korsakov's syndrome is also believed to result from thiamine deficiency, although a similar condition may occur after head injury. It may be a sequel of delirium tremens or Wernicke's encephalopathy. Haemorrhage, necrosis and gliosis are present in the mammillary bodies and hippocampus. There is a gross defect of short-term memory, with consequent disorientation, and some patients attempt to compensate by confabulation. Peripheral neuropathy is often associated with Korsakov's syndrome.

Thiamine deficiency in these conditions may be demonstrated by finding an abnormally large increase in serum pyruvate after glucose ingestion.

Alcoholic dementia leads to a global impairment of mental functions, often accompanied by personality changes of the type caused by frontal lobe damage. CT scan may show cerebral atrophy, which is partly reversible if the patient stops drinking.

Epilepsy may develop because of the direct toxicity of alcohol, especially if there is pre-existing cerebral damage; alcohol withdrawal; overhydration; or hypoglycaemia. Ten per cent of alcoholics have fits.

Neuropathy is a result of thiamine deficiency, and affects motor, sensory, and autonomic nerves. It may present with impotence or with burning pain in the feet.

Other neurological complications (Pearce, 1977) include cerebellar degeneration, central pontine myelinosis, degeneration of the corpus callosum, retrobulbar neuritis, and subdural haematoma following falls.

Drug interactions include potentiation of cerebral depressants; alteration of the rate of metabolism of other drugs, e.g. phenytoin and warfarin, which are broken down by the same liver enzymes; and the accumulation of alcohol's metabolic products, e.g. acetaldehyde, with drugs which interfere with the breakdown pathway — disulfiram, citrated calcium carbonate, and oral antidiabetic agents.

Alcoholic hallucinosis often starts during a phase of abstinence and recovers spontaneously after a few months. Auditory hallucinations, usually voices, develop in clear consciousness. Some insight may be present, but the voices can form a basis for the development of a delusional system.

Alcoholic paranoia is the development of paranoid delusions in the absence of hallucinations. 'Morbid jealousy' of the patient's sexual partner is a frequent theme.

Alcoholic hallucinosis and alcoholic paranoia may respond to phenothiazines. Their relationship, if any, to paranoid schizophrenia is disputed. They are reviewed by Cutting (1978).

Family life is probably always damaged to some extent. Marital breakdown, and violence towards children or spouse, are common.

Working efficiency is reduced, often leading to demotion or unemployment.

Crime: many alcoholics steal to get money for drink. Intoxication may precipitate violence; about 50% of violent crimes are committed when the offender is drunk. Fifty per cent of men in prison have a drinking problem.

Drunken driving: 80 mg% is the legal upper limit for drivers in the UK; it may be too lenient as driving skills are demonstrably impaired at 30 mg%. One in three drivers killed in accidents is drunk.

Suicide is the cause of death in about 15% of alcoholics. Fifty per cent of non-fatal self-poisonings take place following alcohol consumption.

Course

The pattern of drinking varies considerably, but a typical course of events is as follows.

Controlled alcohol consumption increases for psychological reasons, e.g. social pressures to drink, or the presence of stress from which alcohol provides relief. This stage of psychological dependence is followed by the development of physical dependence, manifest by loss of control over the amount consumed, and withdrawal symptoms (tremor, sweating, anxiety, craving) if alcohol is unavailable for a few hours. Intake increases further to combat withdrawal symptoms. Alcohol tolerance increases initially, but may decrease again when the condition becomes more advanced. Drinking gains priority over other activities so that the patient's life suffers in many spheres, and the various physical, psychiatric, and social complications may ensue.

The patient is likely to deny that any problem exists until the resulting damage is gross. He may conceal the extent of his drinking, and hide bottles at home or work.

Heavy smoking, and heavy gambling, are often associated with alcoholism.

Vagrant (skid row) alcoholics are men without families, homes, money, or jobs, often handicapped by low intelligence or chronic mental illness, who live rough in cities, drinking meths or cider, and getting repeated drunkenness convictions.

Jellinek (1960) described five types of drinking problem:

Alpha:	psychological dependence only
Beta:	physical complications without dependence
Gamma:	physical dependence with loss of control
Delta:	physical dependence with loss of control and inability to abstain without withdrawal symptoms
Epsilon:	bout drinking.

Treatment

There is little point in attempting to treat the many alcoholics who deny their problem, or do not want to stop drinking.

Those who are motivated to stop may be able to do so of their own accord. Others need help both to stop drinking and to cope with any associated problems.

Patients' families may need help too, and it is often desirable to involve them anyway as a source of support to the patient.

Total abstinence was the accepted goal of treatment until it was recently noted that some alcoholics had successfully reverted to controlled social drinking, and suggested that this might be an alternative (Pattison, 1976). The indications for aiming at controlled drinking remain to be evaluated, but it would seem a reasonable goal for those who would prefer it to total abstinence, and who do not have cirrhosis or other physical complications which would make any further alcohol consumption dangerous.

Methods of treatment include:

1. *Psychotherapy:* this may be either dynamic or supportive, individual or group, inpatient or outpatient. Inpatient alcoholic units offer intensive group psychotherapy over a few weeks or months. Alcoholics Anonymous provides long-term supportive group therapy at evening meetings, and also runs groups for the spouses and children of alcoholics.

2. *Drugs:* disulfiram (Antabuse) blocks the action of acetaldehyde dehydrogenase, so that there is an accumulation of acetaldehyde if alcohol is combined with it. The combination can produce cardiac arrhythmias or extreme hypotension, sometimes fatal. Side-effects of disulfiram include tiredness, depression, halitosis, gastrointestinal upset, frequency of micturition, peripheral neuritis, impotence, breathlessness, dermatitis, and confusion. It may be given as tablets or an implant. It should only be used in those who appreciate the risk of combining it with alcohol, and require an extra deterrant to reinforce an existing resolve. Citrated calcium carbonate (Abstem) is a similar but safer drug.

3. *Behaviour therapy:* aversion therapy, giving an unpleasant stimulus (e.g. an electric shock or a drug to produce nausea) in combination with alcohol, was once used but is now disfavoured for ethical reasons. The behavioural methods currently employed include teaching alternative ways of reducing anxiety, and methods of controlling the amount of alcohol consumption.

4. *Detoxification only:* detoxification, using medical treatment as outlined for delirium tremens, may be necessary as a prelude to one of the treatments above, but may also be used alone to get the patient over the initial hurdle of stopping regular heavy drinking. Special detoxification centres were recently opened in some areas, and those found drunk in public treated there rather than in the police cells.

It has not been proved that any treatment improves the prognosis, or that one method is superior to another (Orford and Edwards, 1977). The strength of the patient's resolve to stop drinking may be the most important factor influencing outcome.

Provision of long-term support is welcomed by many patients. This may comprise a follow-up group, or residence in a hostel for ex-alcoholics.

Prognosis

About 30% of patients remain abstinent, and another 30% show some improvement, following a course of treatment in an alcoholic unit and subsequent outpatient groups. Such patients have usually been selected as being likely to benefit from intensive treatment and would probably have had a good prognosis anyway.

If relapses occur, they are usually within a few weeks of leaving treatment.

Poor prognostic factors are female sex, youth, poor premorbid personality, and social isolation.

Prevention (Royal College of Psychiatrists, 1979)

A reduction in national per capita alcohol consumption, and hence a reduction in the number of people with alcohol-related problems, could be achieved by:

1. increasing the price of alcohol.
2. reducing availability of alcohol by stopping supermarket sales and retaining licensing laws.
3. discouraging the provision of alcohol as an integral part of business and social functions.
4. banning advertisements for drinks.
5. education about the dangers of alcohol in schools and through the 'media'.

References

Cutting, J. (1978). A reappraisal of alcoholic psychoses. *Psychol. Med.*, **8**, 285–296.

Jellinek, E. M. (1960). *The Disease Concept of Alcoholism*. Hillhouse Press, New Jersey.

Orford, J., and Edwards, G. (1977). *Alcoholism*. Oxford University Press, Oxford.

Pattison, E. M. (1976). Nonabstinent drinking goals in the treatment of alcoholism. *Arch. Gen. Psychiatry*, **33**, 923-931.

Pearce, J. M. S. (1977). Neurological aspects of alcoholism. *Br. J. Hosp. Med.*, **18**, 132-142.

Royal College of Psychiatrists (1979). *Alcohol and Alcoholism*. Tavistock, London.

Shields, J. (1977). Genetics and alcoholism. In *Alcoholism; New Knowledge and New Responses* (Eds. G. Edwards and M. Grant). Croon Helm, London.

World Health Organization (1952). *Expert Committee on Mental Health, Alcoholism Subcommittee, Second Report*. Technical Report Series No. 48. WHO, Geneva.

CHAPTER 10

Drug Abuse

Definitions

Abuse: use of drugs outside the social, medical, or legal norms.

Dependence: defined by WHO (1969) as 'a state, psychic and sometimes also physical, resulting from the interaction between a living organism and a drug, characterised by behavioural and other responses that always include a compulsion to take the drug on a continuous or periodic basis in order to experience its psychic effects, and sometimes to avoid the discomfort of its absence. Tolerance may or may not be present'.

Psychological dependence is a strong desire to take the drug to produce pleasure or relieve distress, and physical dependence is indicated by the development of physical symptoms if the drug is withdrawn. The two types of dependence may be impossible to distinguish.

Tolerance: a state of physical adaptation leading to a diminished response to the same dose of the drug, and so to the need for increasingly large doses to produce the same effect. Tolerance often precedes the development of physical dependence.

Addiction: the use of drugs with detrimental results on social, physical, or economic functioning.

Epidemiology and Aetiology

1. *Sex:* about four times more common in men.

2. *Age:* highest rates occur during adolescence.

3. *Psychological and social factors:* these are important as indicated by the frequency of:
   (a) disturbed family background.
   (b) history of antisocial behaviour.
   (c) drug-taking among other members of the patient's social group.

4. *Genetic predisposition:* has not been demonstrated.

Drugs which invite abuse include cerebral depressants, cerebral stimulants and hallucinogens. Many drug abusers take a mixture of drugs, the choice depending on availability, price, and fashion as well as pharmacology.

The Misuse of Drugs Act, 1971, governs the production, distribution, prescribing, and possession of certain drugs. The drugs controlled under this Act are divided into Classes A, B, and C, Class A drugs being considered most dangerous and carrying the most severe penalties for misuse.

The effects of some individual drugs will be described. Alcohol abuse was described in Chapter 9.

Opiates

Opiates include opium, morphine, heroin, methadone, pethidine, and dipipanone. Opium and morphine are derived from the opium poppy, the others can be synthesized chemically.

Legal status and availability: opiates are Class A drugs. Most addicts obtain their supplies on the black market. There are also 5000 registered addicts in Britain: this number has recently increased by 20% per year. The drugs can be prescribed to relieve severe pain and some 'iatrogenic' addicts are created as a result.

Administration: usually intravenous, but may be by any route.

Psychological and social effects: acute; intravenous injection may produce either intense pleasure or malaise. Chronic; apathy, moodiness, and clouding of consciousness. Most addicts' social circumstances deteriorate, and the need to obtain the drug dominates their lives.

Physical effects: nausea, constipation, constricted pupils. Large doses cause respiratory depression. Infections (abscesses, phlebitis, septicaemia, hepatitis, pneumonia) from unsterile injections are common.

Tolerance and dependence: greatly increased tolerance, and physical dependence, develop within a few weeks of regular use. Endorphin neurotransmitters are probably involved. There is a severe withdrawal syndrome consisting of craving, sleepiness, rhinorrhoea, lacrimation, abdominal colic, and diarrhoea.

Detection: opiates can be detected by blood and urine tests.

Treatment: opiate addicts should be notified to the Home Office and their prescriptions issued only by a doctor with a special licence, working from a treatment centre. Methadone, which is taken orally, is usually prescribed for maintenance.

Prognosis: some opiate addicts give up their drugs either spontaneously or with specialized help. Mortality is increased about 15 times, the most frequent causes of death being respiratory depression from drug overdose, infections, and suicide.

Barbiturates

Legal status and availability: barbiturates are not controlled drugs but their prescription is discouraged. There are still many older people who are dependent on barbiturates which had been prescribed to them as hypnotics. Barbiturates are also used by young drug takers.

Administration: oral or intravenous.

Psychological effects: CNS depression causing psychomotor impairment, drowsiness, or sleep depending on the dose.

Physical effects: ataxia, nystagmus, slurred speech. Respiratory depression occurs with overdoses, which may therefore be fatal. Cross-tolerance with alcohol and anaesthetics occurs.

Tolerance and dependence: tolerance and physical dependence develop rapidly. There is a withdrawal syndrome of anxiety, insomnia, tremor, fits, and delirium.

Detection: barbiturates can be detected by blood and urine tests.

Amphetamines

Legal status and availability: injectable amphetamines are Class A, and oral amphetamines Class B drugs. They used to be prescribed for depression and obesity, and many middle-aged women consequently became dependent. There is now a voluntary ban on prescription, but amphetamines are easily synthesized and so widely used by young drug takers.

Administration: oral or intravenous.

Psychological effects: amphetamines are stimulants which cause euphoria, increased activity, insomnia, and anorexia. 'Amphetamine psychosis' (Connell, 1958) may be caused by repeated use, and consists of visual or auditory hallucinations with paranoid delusions. It is similar to paranoid schizophrenia, but nearly always recovers within a week if the drug is withdrawn.

Physical effects: symptoms of sympathetic nervous system overactivity.

Tolerance and dependence: psychological dependence and tolerance occur. It is not certain whether physical dependence does.

Detection: amphetamines can be detected by blood and urine tests.

Cocaine

Cocaine is derived from the coca shrub which grows in S. America.

Legal status and availability: cocaine is a Class A drug. It is not used in medical practice, and supplies for addicts are imported from S. America.

Administration: inhaled as snuff, drunk in wine, or injected sub-cutaneously.

Psychological and physical effects: similar to those of amphetamine. The 'cocaine psychosis' differs from the amphetamine psychosis in that it often includes tactile hallucinations consisting of a sensation of insects crawling on the skin ('formication'). Inhalation of cocaine may cause perforation of the nasal septum.

Tolerance and dependence: psychological dependence occurs. Tolerance and physical dependence probably do not.

Detection: cocaine can be detected by blood and urine tests.

Treatment: addicts must be notified to the Home Office. Maintenance prescriptions can only be issued by doctors with a special licence.

Cannabis (Indian Hemp, Hashish)

Cannabis is the name given to products of the plant *Cannabis sativa*, which include hashish and marihuana. The active ingredient is tetrahydrocannabinol (THC). *Cannabis sativa* grows wild in Britain and many other countries. THC can also be chemically synthesized.

Legal status and availability: cannabis is a Class B drug, but is freely available from unofficial sources and is probably used by at least 10% of young people in this country. It is often suggested that it could be legalized as it has few adverse effects.

Administration: it is usually mixed with tobacco and smoked, but can also be taken orally or intravenously.

Psychological and social effects: acute; cannabis usually causes well-being, relaxation, and sociability, but it can exaggerate an unpleasant pre-existing mood state of anger, depression, or anxiety. Perceptual distortions and sometimes visual hallucinations occur. Precipitation of psychosis happens very occasionally. Chronic; apathy, lowered efficiency and dementia have been reported in Eastern countries after long-term use, but are unproven.

Physical effects: acute; mild physiological changes, e.g. tachycardia, may occur. Cannabis is an antiemetic and has been successfully used to treat nausea associated with cytotoxic drug treatment. Chronic; only those of the associated tobacco smoking.

Tolerance and dependence: psychological dependence is common, but tolerance and physical dependence do not occur.

Detection: cannabis cannot be detected by routine laboratory tests.

Prognosis: cannabis use appears harmless in most cases. There is no evidence that it predisposes directly to the use of more dangerous drugs, except through encouraging social contact with other drug users.

Lysergic Acid Diethylamide (LSD)

LSD is a synthetic compound.

Legal status and availability: LSD, a Class A drug, is not currently used in medical practice in the UK, but can easily be synthesized by amateur chemists.

Administration: oral.

Psychological effects: perceptual distortion, abreaction of distant memories, extreme depression or ecstasy ('bad trips' or 'good trips'). 'Flashbacks' of similar experiences may occur up to a year after the last dose. LSD may precipitate psychosis.

Physical effects: those of sympathetic nervous system overactivity.

Tolerance and dependence: these do not occur.

Detection: LSD cannot be detected by routine laboratory tests.

Glues and Solvents

Fumes from products based on toluene and acetone have been increasingly used for their psychological effects in recent years. Such products include glues and solvents for domestic or industrial use. They are freely available and are popular among children.

Administration: inhalation from paper, bottle, or bag ('glue-sniffing').

Psychological effects: euphoria and perceptual disturbance, progressing to stupor.

Physical effects: the substances are toxic to the liver, kidney, heart, and brain, and inhalation may cause accidental death.

Tolerance and dependence: psychological dependence is common, but tolerance and physical dependence probably do not occur.

Tobacco

Nicotine is probably the constituent of tobacco which causes psychological effects and dependence, whereas carbon monoxide and tar cause the physical ill-effects. Cigarette smoking is more harmful than other forms of tobacco consumption. It is widespread among patients and staff in psychiatric hospitals, despite its ill-effects.

Psychological effects: nicotine is a central nervous system stimulant and an anxiolytic.

Physical effects: acute; those of sympathetic nervous system over-activity. Chronic; raised susceptibility to lung cancer, ischaemic heart disease, chronic bronchitis and, during pregnancy, stillbirth or abortion.

Tolerance and dependence: both psychological and physical dependence occur. There is a withdrawal syndrome consisting of anxiety, depression, irritability, insomnia, and craving, with changes in the EEG and physiological measurements.

Treatment: nicotine chewing-gum is a less toxic alternative which may be an effective aid to giving up smoking. It would be desirable to prevent people from starting to smoke through educational means, or by increasing the price of cigarettes.

Caffeine

Caffeine is a constituent of coffee, tea, cocoa, and cola drinks. It is a xanthine alkaloid.

Psychological effects: caffeine is a stimulant which increases well-being and reduces fatigue. Large doses cause anxiety and insomnia.

Physical effects: tachycardia, diuresis, muscle tension.

Tolerance and dependence: psychological dependence occurs, but not physical dependence.

Caffeine is probably not harmful in the quantities most people consume.

Treatment of Drug Abuse

Treatment of drug abuse will only succeed with the patient's cooperation and motivation. If physical dependence is present, the first stage of treatment is drug withdrawal, often best carried out in hospital. Withdrawal symptoms are avoided by stopping the drug gradually, or substituting another less harmful drug which has cross-tolerance with the original, e.g. methadone for heroin addicts.

The long-term aim of treatment may be either abstinence from drugs, or controlled drug use. Many patients have social problems or personality problems which require extensive and prolonged help. A minority of addicts receive treatment in residential units. Such units are run on therapeutic community lines and require members to abstain from drugs completely. Other patients attend special outpatient clinics for controlled drug supplies.

There are no accurate statistics on outcome of treatment, and no evidence that active treatment can cure addiction. Prevention would be better.

Further Reading

Accounts of drug abuse and its treatment are given by Hofmann and Hofmann (1975), Glatt (1977) and Madden (1979).

References

Connell, P. H. (1958). *Amphetamine Psychosis*. Maudsley Monograph No. 5. Oxford University Press, Oxford.

Glatt, M. M. (Ed.) (1977). *Drug Dependence. Current Problems and Issues*. MTP Press, Lancaster.

Hofmann, F. G., and Hofmann, A. D. (1975). *A Handbook on Drug and Alcohol Abuse*. Oxford University Press, Oxford.

Madden, J. S. (1979). *A Guide to Alcohol and Drug Dependence*. Wright, Bristol.

World Health Organization (1969). *Report of Expert Committee on Addiction-Producing Drugs*. WHO Technical Report Series 407, 11.

CHAPTER 11

Deliberate Self-harm

Deliberate self-harm includes suicide, and non-fatal deliberate self-poisoning or self-injury. These are described separately although there is some overlap between them.

SUICIDE

Definition

An act of self-injury undertaken with conscious self-destructive intent, with a fatal outcome.

Statistics

The suicide rate in England and Wales is about 8 per 100,000 population per year; 4000 cases per year. The rate decreased during the 1960s, was stable in the early 1970s, but is now rising. Official statistics probably underestimate the rate as only deaths with proven evidence of intent are given suicide verdicts by the coroner.

Methods

Poisoning accounts for about 50% of cases. Prescribed psychotropic drugs are the most frequent poisons used. Hanging, shooting, laceration, drowning, and gassing each account for a smaller proportion. The availability of a method influences the frequency with which it is used.

Epidemiology and Aetiology

1. *Age:* the rate increases with age.

2. *Sex:* the male:female ratio is 3:2, but the proportion of cases in women is increasing.

3. *Marital status:* the divorced have the highest rates, followed by the widowed and single, and the married the lowest.

4. *Psychiatric illness:* present immediately before death in about 90% of cases (Barraclough *et al.*, 1974). Depressive illness, often inadequately treated, is the commonest diagnosis, alcoholism next.

The percentage of psychiatric cases who die by suicide is estimated as:

Depressive illness (including both depressive psychosis and depressive neurosis)	15%
Alcoholism	15%
Schizophrenia	10%
Opiate addition	10%
Sociopathy	5%

5. *Physical illness.*

6. *Living alone.*

7. *Unemployment.*

8. *Nationality:* there are large differences between the suicide rates of different countries. Countries with high rates include Austria, Denmark, Japan, and W. Germany; countries with low rates include Ireland, Italy, and the Netherlands.

9. *Urban living:* areas of big cities with a mobile population have high rates.

10. *National circumstances:* the rate falls in wartime, and rises in times of economic depression.

11. *Social class:* highest rates in class I, followed by classes II and V.

12. *Season:* highest rates in the spring, perhaps because of the increase of depressive illness then.

Durkheim (1894) postulated that 'anomie', a sense of isolation from the community, was contributory to suicide, and many of the above observations support this theory.

Prevention

Preventive strategies are difficult to evaluate because so many factors affect the suicide rate. Suggested measures include:

1. *Improved training for GPs* and others in diagnosis and treatment of depression and other psychiatric illness.

2. *Restricting availability* of potentially lethal drugs, gases, and weapons.

3. *Counselling services* such as the Samaritan organization.

NON-FATAL DELIBERATE SELF-HARM
(DSH, PARASUICIDE, ATTEMPTED SUICIDE)

Definition

An act in which an individual deliberately causes self-injury or ingests a substance in excess of any prescribed or generally recognized therapeutic dose, without a fatal outcome.

Incidence

About 120,000 cases annually in England and Wales. The rate has increased since the 1950s. Self-poisoning is the commonest reason for admission to a medical ward for young people.

Methods

Over 90% of cases are self-poisonings and the rest mostly self-lacerations. Psychotropic drugs are the most frequent poisons used, and proprietary analgesics next. Alcohol is taken at the same time in about 50% of cases.

Epidemiology and Aetiology

1. *Age:* the rate is highest in the late teens and early twenties.

2. *Sex:* the male:female ratio is about 1:2. Young age groups have the greatest excess of women.

3. *Psychiatric abnormality:*

Depression	50–60%
Alcoholism	10–20%
Personality disorder	15–30%
None	10–20%

4. *Social conditions:* highest rates are in social classes IV and V, and in city areas where there is a high incidence of social problems.

5. *Life events:* about 70% of acts follow a distressing event, usually involving disharmony with another person.

Motives

About 10% of episodes are serious suicide attempts which fail. In other cases the reported motivation is commonly escape from an intolerable situation or state of mind, an appeal for help, or an attempt to influence another person, but some patients cannot explain their motivation.

Assessment

1. Whether there was serious suicidal intent, as indicated by:
   (a) the patient claiming to have wanted to die and regret survival.
   (b) a premeditated act preceded by making arrangements for death, leaving a suicide note, and taking precautions against discovery.
   (c) use of a method which the patient believed would be fatal.
   (d) the presence of characteristics associated with completed suicide.
2. Whether psychiatric illness requiring treatment is present.
3. Whether remediable social problems are present.

Assessment by a psychiatrist is officially recommended for all cases, but deliberate self-harm is now so frequent that this poses practical problems. Trials indicate that junior medical staff, nurses, and social workers, with appropriate training, are quite competent to select those cases needing psychiatric care.

Management

About 20% of cases require psychiatric hospital admission because of psychiatric illness and/or continuing suicidal intentions. About 50% are judged to need psychiatric and/or social work follow-up, although a high proportion default.

Prognosis

About 20% repeat deliberate self-harm in the subsequent year, 1% die by suicide in the subsequent year and 10% probably die by suicide eventually.

Prevention

1. *Psychiatric treatment*, social work or counselling have not been shown to reduce the repetition rate for deliberate self-harm, although they are valuable for some associated problems.

2. *Restricting availability* of psychotropic drugs and analgesics might reduce the number of impulsive overdoses.

Further Reading

Books on deliberate self-harm include those by Farmer and Hirsch (1980), Morgan (1979), and Stengel (1964), and a booklet by the Office of Health Economics (1981). The book by Kreitman (1977) deals with non-fatal cases only.

References

Barraclough, B. M., Bunch, J., Nelson, B., and Sainsbury, P. (1974). A hundred cases of suicide: clinical aspects. *Br. J. Psychiatry* **125**, 355–373.

Durkheim, E. (1894). *Suicide*. Trans. J. A. Spaulding and G. Simpson. (1952) Routledge and Kegan Paul, London.

Farmer, R. D. and Hirsch, S. R. (Eds.) (1980). *The Suicide Syndrome*. Croon Helm, London.

Kreitman, N. (Ed.) (1977). *Parasuicide*. Wiley, Chichester.

Morgan, H. G. (1979). *Death Wishes? The Understanding and Management of Deliberate Self-Harm*. Wiley, Chichester.

Office of Health Economics (1981). *Suicide and Deliberate Self-Harm*. OHE, London.

Stengel, E. (1964). *Suicide and Attempted Suicide*. Penguin, Harmondsworth.

CHAPTER 12

Sexual Disorders

SEXUAL INADEQUACY

Types

Male: Erectile impotence
              Premature ejaculation
              Failure of ejaculation

Female: Vaginismus
              Dyspareunia
              Absence of orgasm

Aetiology

1. *Psychological factors in otherwise normal people*, e.g. anxiety or ignorance about sex, general disharmony between the couple concerned.

2. *Psychiatric illness:* all psychiatric illnesses except mania tend to reduce sexual drive and performance. This is especially true of depressive illnesses and anxiety states.

3. *Organic conditions:*

    (a) genital malformation due to congenital abnormality or trauma.
    (b) neurological or vascular conditions, e.g. peripheral neuropathy, multiple sclerosis, spinal injury, pelvic surgery or irradiation.
    (c) endocrine and metabolic conditions, e.g. diabetes, acromegaly, testosterone deficiency, hyperprolactinaemia, and renal failure.
    (d) aging.
    (e) drugs: hypotensives, sex hormones, opiates, disulfiram, and many psychotropic drugs. Both tricyclic antidepressants and MAOIs can cause

impotence or failure of ejaculation because of their anticholinergic and antiadrenergic effects. Neuroleptics, especially thioridazine, can also cause failure of ejaculation and they may cause loss of libido, impotence, amenorrhoea, and infertility due to increased prolactin secretion.

(f) alcohol abuse: impotence in alcoholics may result from intoxication, peripheral neuropathy, disturbed sex hormone metabolism due to cirrhosis of the liver, or disulfiram treatment.

Treatment

1. *Psychiatric illness or organic pathology* should be given appropriate treatment.

2. *Psychological approaches*, if organic causes and psychiatric illness have been excluded:

(a) simple explanation and counselling is often all that is required, and sometimes this can be provided from books.

(b) behaviour therapy, in which the couple are treated jointly by a pair of cotherapists. This is based on the methods of Masters and Johnson (1970). Treatment begins with a 'sensate focus phase' during which intercourse is not attempted, but the couple spend a set time each day stroking each other's non-genital areas; this is designed to reduce anxiety and improve communication. They are then taught special techniques according to the type of dysfunction present, e.g. the 'squeeze technique' for treatment of premature ejaculation.

(c) psychodynamic psychotherapy if there are complex underlying emotional problems.

3. *Drugs:*

(a) testosterone increases sexual responsiveness in women, but not in men unless a demonstrable testosterone deficiency is present.

(b) bromocriptine may cure impotence secondary to hyperprolactinaemia.

4. *Mechanical aids*, e.g. splints or plastic surgery for impotence, vaginal dilators for vaginismus.

Further Reading

The treatment of sexual dysfunction is described by Gillan and Gillan (1976) and Haslam (1978).

SEXUAL DEVIATIONS

Sexual deviations are sexual practices which are unacceptable to the society concerned. All types are more common in men than in women.

Aetiology

This is unknown, but the following factors have been investigated:

1. *Organic:* a genetic component probably exists in homosexuality, but has not been found in other deviations. No consistent abnormalities of sex hormone secretion have been found, although hormone imbalance in the prenatal period has been suggested, and the sex chromosomes are almost always normal.

2. *Psychodynamic:* many patients describe abnormal parental attitudes, e.g. excessive dominance of one parent, or a desire by the parents for a child of the opposite sex.

3. *Behavioural:* deviant sexual behaviour may be learned by conditioning or modelling, and continued because it reduces anxiety.

Treatment

The aim of treatment may be either to discourage the deviation or, if it is not harmful to others, to help the subject adapt to it. Treatment is only given if the subject wants it, and sexual offenders should not be treated against their will. The following approaches are used.

1. *Psychodynamic psychotherapy*, to explore possible origins of the sexual deviation in disturbed relationships or repressed events in childhood.

2. *Behaviour therapy*, e.g. covert sensitization or aversion therapy to discourage undesirable behaviour, assertive training to increase confidence in heterosexual relationships.

3. *Drugs:*

(a) antilibidinal drugs for male sexual offenders. These include cyproterone acetate, which reduces gonadotrophin release and blocks androgen receptors, benperidol which is a butyrophenone, and oestrogens. They may cause impotence, infertility, and mammary hypertrophy, and so they should only be used for dangerous sexual offenders and with the subject's informed consent.

(b) sex hormones may be used to help transsexuals to resemble a member of the opposite sex. Hormones are not effective in changing sexual orientation.

4. *Surgery:* sex reassignment may help transsexuals. Castration is an effective treatment for sex offenders, but is not used in this country because of ethical objections.

Some types of sexual deviation will be described.

Male Homosexuality (Bancroft, 1970)

Homosexuality, or erotic attachment towards members of the same sex, is common in men. Kinsey *et al.* (1948) found that 4% of American men were exclusively homosexual, and 37% had had some homosexual experience. Since the Sexual Offences Act 1967, homosexual acts carried out in private between men over 21 have not been illegal in Britain.

Most homosexuals have a masculine physical appearance, but a few are effeminate in dress or manner. Homosexuals have higher than normal rates of depression, alcoholism, and neurotic illness, probably because of the stigma still attached to the condition. Those who have some heterosexual interest may marry, but the marriages are seldom successful.

Treatment should only be attempted for those who wish to become heterosexual, or who have associated psychiatric problems. A change of orientation is unusual unless there has been some spontaneous heterosexual interest at some time. Psychotherapy or behaviour therapy may be used, and about 40% of subjects treated by either method improve.

Female Homosexuality (Lesbianism) (Kenyon, 1970)

Lesbianism is less common than male homosexuality, being present in about 2% of women. Subjects probably have an increased prevalence of personality disorders and neurotic symptoms, but they seldom seek treatment for their homosexuality. Lesbianism has never been illegal.

Transvestism (Randell, 1970)

Transvestism is a wish or compulsion to wear clothing of the opposite sex. It usually begins in childhood. Cross-dressing is often associated with sexual arousal. Almost all transvestites are male, and most are heterosexual, but sometimes the condition is associated with homosexuality, transsexualism, or other sexual deviations.

Transvestism is common, and is not illegal. It only comes to psychiatric attention if the subject or his wife is concerned about it, or if there is a compulsion to cross-dress in public.

Transsexualism (Schapira, 1979)

Transsexualism is a disorder of gender identity in which there is a wish to change to the opposite sex, with a conviction of having been born into the wrong sex, present since early childhood. About 80% of transsexuals are male. Many are married with children, but a few are homosexual.

Few transsexuals wish to live as a member of their biological sex, and treatment to reconcile them to this is unlikely to work. They often request surgical sex reassignment. The present criteria for this operation are that the subject has firmly and consistently asked for it, has lived as a member of the opposite sex for one to two years with the aid of hormone therapy, is currently unmarried, and is psychologically stable. Most cases who fulfil these criteria are pleased with the results of surgery. The operation is combined with hormone treatment to change the secondary sex characteristics, and tuition in behaviour appropriate to the new sex.

Exhibitionism (Indecent Exposure) (Rooth, 1980)

Exhibitionism is exposure of the genitals to another person, usually carried out by a man in the presence of a girl or women who is unknown to him. It is illegal, but many offenders do not try to avoid detection and expose repeatedly in the same place. They seldom rape or even touch the victim.

Most exhibitionists are young men who have poor sexual adjustment. Some are anxious, inhibited men who feel guilty about exposing, others are sociopathic men who derive pleasure and excitement from it. If a man exposes for the first time in middle or old age, an underlying condition such as psychotic illness, dementia, or frontal lobe damage should be excluded.

Victims of exposure may be temporarily distressed, but seldom suffer serious emotional consequences.

Incest (Bluglass, 1979)

Incest is sexual intercourse with a parent, sibling, child, or grandchild, and is an imprisonable offence. The most common forms are between father and daughter, and between brother and sister. It is commonly associated with overcrowding and poor social conditions, or occurs in families in which the parents' sexual relationship is poor. Some girls involved in incestuous relationships have sexual difficulties in later life, but the frequency of long-term ill-effects is unknown. It is thought that there is a greatly increased rate of genetic defects in children born as a result of incest.

Paedophilia

Paedophilia is a sexual preference for prepubertal children, and is an imprisonable offence.

It occurs in men, and less often in women, who have difficulty forming sexual relationships with adults, and varies from an affectionate relationship with a known child to the homicidal rape of a strange one. Homosexual and heterosexual types exist. Dangerous paedophiliacs require secure care and antilibidinal drugs.

Sadism and Masochism

Sadism is sexual gratification which involves inflicting cruelty on the partner. Masochism, which often exists in the same individual, is a related condition in which sexual gratification involves being subjected to cruelty. Minor forms of both conditions are common. Extreme forms of sadism may lead to sexual crimes.

Fetishism

Fetishism is the condition in which a part of the body other than the genitals, or an inanimate object, is the main object of sexual desire. It can often be explained by a learned association between the fetish object and sexual arousal, and can be treated by behaviour therapy.

Voyeurism

Voyeurism is sexual gratification through watching the sexual activity of others. It is often associated with other sexual deviations, but is not associated with more serious sexual offences.

Bestiality

Bestiality is intercourse with animals. It is most common in male adolescent farm workers, and is illegal.

Rape

Rape is described in Chapter 15.

References

Bancroft, J. H. J. (1970). Homosexuality in the male. *Br. J. Hosp. Med.*, **3**, 168–181.

Bluglass, R. (1979). Incest. *Br. J. Hosp. Med.*, **22**, 152–157.

Gillan, P., and Gillan, R. (1976). *Sex Therapy Today*. Open Books, London.

Haslam, M. T. (1978). *Sexual Disorders*. Pitman, London.

Kenyon, F. E. (1970). Homosexuality in the female. *Br. J. Hosp. Med.*, **3**, 183–206.

Kinsey, A. C., Pomeroy, W. B., and Martin, C. E. (1948). *Sexual Behaviour in the Human Male*. Saunders, Philadelphia.

Masters, W. H., and Johnson, V. E. (1970). *Human Sexual Inadequacy*. Little, Brown, Boston.

Randell, J. (1970). Transvestism and trans sexualism. *Br. J. Hosp. Med.*, **3**, 211–213.

Rooth, G. (1980). Exhibitionism: an eclectic approach to its management. *Br. J. Hosp. Med.*, **23**, 366–370.

Schapira, K. (1979). The assessment and management of transsexual problems. *Br. J. Hosp. Med.* **22**, 63–69.

CHAPTER 13

Disorders of Childbearing

PUERPERAL PSYCHOSIS

Definition

A psychosis beginning within 12 weeks of delivery.

Incidence

Following 1 in 500 births.

Predisposing Factors

1. *Past history of psychosis.*

2. *Family history of psychosis.*

3. *Primiparity.*

4. *Stressful circumstances surrounding pregnancy or birth.*

Aetiology

1. The delirium so often present when the illness starts suggests an organic cause, but the hormone changes which have been suggested as an obvious one have not been found to differ from those which take place in all post-partum women.
2. Childbirth may be a non-specific stress precipitating illness in women already predisposed.

Clinical Features

Premonitory symptoms may occur in late pregnancy, but onset of frank psychosis is usually sudden, 2–14 days after delivery. The initial picture often has the features of delirium, and a few cases do turn out to be toxic confusional states due to pelvic infection, but usually the delirious features subside in a few days and symptoms of one of the functional psychoses appear. The order of frequency is depressive psychosis, schizophrenia, and mania. The thought content, and any delusions or hallucinations present, usually concern the baby, with a risk of infanticide.

Treatment

Hospital admission is usually necessary, preferably to a unit where mother and baby may be kept together under supervision to encourage 'bonding' between them.

Treatment is the same as would be used for the equivalent psychosis occurring apart from the puerperium. If appropriate, ECT is often used in preference to drugs, since drugs enter breast milk.

Prognosis

Short-term prognosis is very good, but there is a 20% chance of recurrence after any subsequent pregnancy, and a 50% chance of later recurrence not related to pregnancy.

ATYPICAL DEPRESSION AFTER CHILDBIRTH (Pitt 1968)

Incidence

Following 1 in 10 births.

Predisposing Factors

1. *Neurotic traits* in the premorbid personality.

Aetiology

1. *Psychological difficulties* in accepting motherhood, coping with the added responsibilities and the changed social role.

2. *Minor hormonal imbalance* could be contributory but has not been demonstrated.

Clinical Features

Mild depression, anxiety, fatigue, loss of libido, anorexia, and insomnia, which may last for months or years.

Treatment

1. *Drugs:* tricyclic antidepressants or monoamine oxidase inhibitors.

2. *Psychotherapy:* individual, family, or group.

3. *Training in child care* and introduction to groups of other mothers of young children may help. Such measures in pregnancy might have prophylactic value.

ABORTION

The Abortion Act 1967 legalized abortion before 28 weeks of pregnancy if, in the opinion of two doctors, one or more of the following conditions applied:

1. risk to the life of the mother would be greater if the pregnancy were continued rather than terminated.
2. risk to the mental or physical health of the mother would be greater if the pregnancy were continued rather than terminated.
3. a risk to the health of existing children would be present if the pregnancy were continued.
4. there would be a substantial risk of the child having a mental or physical handicap.

The Act has been criticized for being so loosely worded that it permits abortion on demand, which was not its intention.

Sixty per cent of abortions are done on psychiatric grounds, but usually without specialized psychiatric advice.

Post-partum psychosis after a previous delivery is usually regarded as a justification for abortion if the woman wants one, but since risk of recurrent post-partum psychosis after a single previous episode is only 20%, abortion should not be advised automatically. The risk of an equivalent psychosis being precipitated by abortion is very small.

Abortion seldom has serious psychiatric sequelae (Greer *et al.*, 1976). About 25% of women experience some guilt or depression afterwards, usually mild and transient. Symptoms are more likely if the woman was uncertain about wanting the abortion or was pressurized to accept it.

Further Reading

Psychiatric aspects of childbirth are reviewed in the book edited by Sandler (1978).

References

Greer, H. S., Lal, S., Lewis, S. C., Belsey, E. M., and Beard, R. W. (1976). Psychosocial consequences of therapeutic abortion. *Br. J. Psychiatry* **128**, 74–79.

Pitt, B. (1968). 'Atypical' depression following childbirth. *Br. J. Psychiatry* **114**, 1325–1335.

Sandler, M. (Ed.) (1978). *Mental Illness in Pregnancy and the Puerperium*. Oxford University Press, Oxford.

CHAPTER 14

Anorexia Nervosa

Definition

Anorexia nervosa is characterized by extreme weight loss achieved by dieting and other means; amenorrhoea, or impotence in males; abnormal attitudes to food; and a distorted body image.

Prevalence (Crisp *et al.*, 1976)

Up to 1% of adolescent girls are affected. The prevalence appears to be increasing, and mild partial versions of the syndrome are common.

Epidemiology

1. *Age:* most cases start in adolescence, occasional ones in childhood or adult life.

2. *Sex:* 95% are female.

3. *Social class:* classes I and II predominate.

Clinical Features

Physical: the patient loses weight by dietary restriction, especially of carbohydrates, and sometimes by self-induced vomiting, taking laxatives or diuretics, and excessive exercising. Amenorrhoea occurs, sometimes before there has been much loss of weight. In male patients there is loss of sexual interest and impotence. Other common physical features are hypotension, bradycardia, constipation, mild hypothermia, and a growth of downy (lanugo) hair. Vomiting or purging may result in disturbance of fluid and electrolyte balance.

Mental: the patient is preoccupied with food and weight, takes pride in dieting, and feels guilty about eating more than a small amount. Most patients do not see themselves as unwell or underweight, but feel active, healthy, and fashionably slim. Some, however, especially those in whom the condition has become chronic, have greater insight and may become severely depressed.

A variant of anorexia nervosa, in which overeating followed by vomiting or purging occurs, is termed 'bulimia nervosa' and has a worse prognosis (Russell, 1979).

Psychodynamic theories view the illness as a means of avoiding maturation, especially in sexual terms; or as a means of acquiring independence and a sense of achievement through strict control of diet and weight. These attitudes may stem from disturbed family relationships, which are always evident in the established case but may be largely a result, not a cause, of the condition.

Endocrine and Metabolic Changes (Russell, 1977)

Hypothalamic dysfunction is always present. It is thought to be secondary to the weight loss, in which case anorexia nervosa could be classed as a 'psychosomatic' disease, but it could be a primary abnormality. Laboratory tests show:

1. reduction of sex hormone, gonadotrophin, and thyroid hormone secretion.
2. increase of growth hormone and cortisol secretion.
3. increased insulin response to glucose loading.
4. low basal temperature and impaired temperature regulation.
5. low basal metabolic rate.
6. high serum cholesterol and blood urea, if there is a high protein intake.

Differential Diagnosis

1. *Chronic debilitating physical disease.*

2. *Psychiatric illnesses:* depression, schizophrenia, obsessional neurosis.

3. *Hypothalamic lesions.*

Treatment (Russell, 1981)

Severe cases require hospital admission, and treatment of any physical complications of malnutrition which are present. Milder cases may be treated as outpatients. The aims of treatment are restoration of normal weight, of normal attitudes towards food, eating, and body size, and resolution of problems in relationships or other spheres of life.

Weight gain is best achieved by obtaining the patient's agreement to eat more. Many patients are reluctant to do so, and may vomit or dispose of food in secret; behaviour therapy, in which privileges are given to reward weight gain, may be used in such cases. Drugs (chlorpromazine, amitriptyline, appetite stimulants, or modified insulin therapy) may help by increasing appetite, decreasing resistance to eating, and treating associated depression. Psychotherapy is an important aspect of treatment, for without a change in the patient's attitudes, any weight gained as a result of hospital treatment will be lost again when the patient goes home.

Leucotomy has been used in chronic severe cases, but may result in uncontrolled eating which distresses the patient.

Prognosis (Morgan and Russell, 1975)

Recovery is judged by return to normal weight, return of menstruation, and improved psychological adjustment. About a third of patients recover fully, a third make a partial recovery, and the rest do badly. About 5% die from suicide or less often from physical complications. Poor prognostic factors are a long history, older age, abnormal premorbid personality, and extreme weight loss.

References

Crisp, A. H., Palmer, R. L., and Kalucy, R. S. (1976). How common is anorexia nervosa? A prevalence study. *Br. J. Psychiatry* **128**, 549–554.

Morgan, H. G., and Russell, G. M. F. (1975). Value of family background and clinical features as predictors of long-term outcome of anorexia nervosa: four-year follow-up study of 41 patients. *Psychol. Med.* **5**, 355–371.

Russell, G. F. M. (1977). Editorial: the present status of anorexia nervosa. *Psychol. Med.* **7**, 363–367.

Russell, G. F. M. (1979). Bulimia nervosa: an ominous variant of anorexia nervosa. *Psychol. Med.* **9**, 429–448.

Russell, G. F. M. (1981). The current treatment of anorexia nervosa. *Br. J. Psychiatry* **138**, 164–166.

CHAPTER 15

Forensic Psychiatry

About 30% of men in prison have a psychiatric disorder of a severity requiring treatment. The commonest diagnoses are sociopathy and alcoholism; there is also an excess of mental subnormality, functional psychosis, organic brain disease, and epilepsy among prisoners. However, social and cultural factors are more important than psychiatric illness in causing crime.

Male prisoners outnumber female ones 30-fold. Cultural factors probably account for most of this discrepancy, but the increased frequency of criminal behaviour among men with the XYY genotype suggests that biological factors also contribute. Female prisoners have more mental and physical disease than male ones.

Murder (Bluglass, 1979)

There are 400–500 murders per year in England and Wales. In 75% of cases the victim is well known to the murderer, most often the spouse. About 50% of murderers have a serious psychiatric abnormality. Many commit suicide after their crime.

The main psychiatric conditions which can lead to murder are:

1. psychoses: a severely depressed person may murder children or other relatives because of a delusion that they are going to suffer a worse fate. Schizophrenics may commit murder under the influence of paranoid delusions. Puerperal psychosis accounts for some, but not all, cases of infanticide.
2. sociopathic personality disorder.
3. drug-induced states.
4. 'morbid jealousy'.
5. mental handicap, in which frustration may be expressed by violence.
6. epileptic automatism: this is a rare cause, and there is no significant association between murder and epilepsy.

About 75% of murderers whose crime was apparently motiveless have an abnormal EEG.

The presence of mental disorder may cause the charge to be reduced from murder to manslaughter on the grounds of diminished responsibility, under the Homicide Act 1957. A verdict of murder always carries a sentence of life imprisonment, but manslaughter may receive any sentence, including a hospital order on Section 60 or 65, or discharge.

Less often, a mentally abnormal offender accused of murder or other serious crime is found 'unfit to plead', and is sent directly to a psychiatric hospital. If he recovers he may be required to stand trial. The grounds for being unfit to plead are: inability to instruct counsel, to appreciate the significance of pleading, to challenge a juror, to examine a witness, or to understand the evidence or court procedure.

A rare plea in murder cases is 'not guilty by reason of insanity', when the offender fulfils the MacNaughten Rules, that is he either did not know the nature and quality of his act, or did not know that it was wrong. A deluded patient is assumed to be under the same degree of responsibility as he would be if the delusions were true. If this plea is successful, the accused is sent to a Special Hospital.

About half those accused of murder claim amnesia for the event, but this is not an adequate defence, nor is drunkenness.

Rape (Gibbens *et al.*, 1977)

Rape is sexual intercourse with a woman without her consent. About 400 rapes are reported annually in England and Wales, but most cases are probably not reported.

The following types of rapist are described:

1. inhibited men who are unable to form normal sexual relationships.
2. aggressive violent men with contempt for women.
3. the psychiatrically ill or mentally handicapped.
4. group rape, by gangs of youths whose members would probably not commit the crime individually.

Of those convicted, 90% do not repeat the crime, but the aggressive type may do so as well as committing other violent crimes, and may require secure care and antilibidinal drugs.

Centres for counselling rape victims have been set up in some cities.

Arson

About 40% of serious fires are started deliberately. Types of arsonist include:

1. those with a criminal motive, e.g. obtaining insurance money or concealing evidence of a crime. They usually have sociopathic personalities.
2. psychotic patients motivated by delusions.
3. those with abnormal personality or low intelligence who start fires for excitement or revenge. They often repeat the offence and require secure detention.

Shoplifting (Gibbens *et al.*, 1971)

Women shoplift more often than men, and shoplifting is the most common crime among female prisoners. A minority of shoplifting episodes are organized crimes. About two-thirds of female shoplifters are depressed middle-aged women. In London's West End, about a third are young foreign women without psychiatric disturbance.

Special Hospitals

Special Hospitals exist for the treatment of psychotic, sociopathic, or mentally handicapped patients who have committed violent crimes. They include Broadmoor, Rampton, Moss Side and Park Lane in England, and Carstairs in Scotland. All patients are compulsorily admitted and detained under the Mental Health Act, the majority from the courts, some from prisons or psychiatric hospitals. Violence to others, violence to self, damage to property, and sex offences are the most frequent reasons for admission. The length of stay is several years but about half the patients are eventually fit for discharge or transfer to conventional psychiatric hospitals.

Some other topics with forensic implications are dealt with in other parts of the book: sexual deviations (Chapter 12), juvenile delinquency and 'baby battering' (Chapter 18), and the Mental Health Act (Chapter 24).

Further Reading

The relationship between psychiatry and crime is reviewed by Gunn (1977).

References

Bluglass, R. (1979). The psychiatric assessment of homicide. *Br. J. Hosp. Med.*, **22**, 366–377.

Gibbens, T. C. N., Palmer, C., and Prince, J. (1971). Mental health aspects of shoplifting. *Br. Med. J.* **3**, 612–615.

Gibbens, T. C. N., Way, C., and Soothill, K. L. (1977). Behavioural types of rape. *Br. J. Psychiatry*, **130**, 32–42.

Gunn, J. (1977). Review Article: Criminal behaviour and mental disorder. *Br. J. Psychiatry*, **130**, 317–329.

CHAPTER 16

Miscellaneous Disorders

This chapter includes some disorders which are not readily classified elsewhere. They are described in alphabetical order.

Amnesia (Whitty, 1978)

Differential diagnosis of amnesia includes:

1. *Psychogenic (hysterical) amnesia:* the patient cannot recall his identity or anything about himself, but can remember information which has no personal relevance to him, and other cognitive functions are intact. Psychogenic amnesia is often associated with a fugue state, in which the patient wanders away from home. There may be an underlying depression, or the amnesia may represent a means of escape from an unpleasant situation, as in those accused of crime. The mental mechanisms of repression and dissociation would explain the phenomenon.

2. *Malingering*, which cannot be reliably differentiated from hysterical amnesia.

3. *Alcohol or drugs.*

4. *Head injury.*

5. *Post-epileptic states.*

6. *Hypoglycaemia.*

7. *Transient global amnesia:* a rare condition occurring in older patients and probably due to impaired cerebral circulation. There is complete amnesia which lasts several hours but then recovers completely.

Bereavement (Parkes, 1965)

Grief after bereavement may last for months and illusions or pseudo-hallucinations of the deceased's presence are not unusual. An abnormal grief reaction may be diagnosed if grieving is unduly prolonged, or if grief cannot be expressed; occasionally there is complete denial that the death has occurred. Bereavement may precipitate depressive illness, other psychiatric illness, or suicide.

Abnormal grief reactions are more common if the deceased was young, if the death was sudden or violent, or if the bereaved person had feelings of guilt or ambivalence about the deceased.

Reactions of a similar kind may follow other kinds of loss like the death of a pet, divorce, loss of a job, or amputation.

If 'biological' depressive symptoms develop after bereavement, they should be treated by drugs or ECT. Psychotherapy may be helpful for some kinds of grief reaction; for instance if expression of grief is inhibited the technique of 'guided mourning', in which the patient is made to confront evidence of the death, has been shown to help.

Capgras Syndrome (Christodoulou, 1977)

The Capgras syndrome (*illusion des sosies*) is the delusional negation of identity of a familiar person. The patient believes that a close relative has been replaced by a double. This rare syndrome occurs in psychotic illness, usually schizophrenia, and most cases have evidence of organic cerebral impairment. Paranoid symptoms, depersonalization and de-realization are often associated with it. Women are affected more often than men.

Ganser Syndrome

The Ganser syndrome consists of giving approximate answers to obvious questions, and clouded consciousness. Impaired memory and attention ('pseudodementia'), hallucinations, and hysterical conversion symptoms are often associated with it. Malingering or hysteria may be the cause, as suggested by the frequency of the syndrome in those accused of crime, and the common impression that the patient has understood the questions. Some cases are secondary to depression or schizophrenia. Spontaneous recovery is usual after a few days.

Gilles de la Tourette's Syndrome

Gilles de la Tourette's syndrome comprises multiple tics and compulsive utterances. Tics develop first in the facial muscles, then spread to other parts of the body. Involuntary utterances then occur, barking noises at first, later obscene words or short phrases (coprolalia). Echolalia and echopraxia may be present.

Onset is usually in childhood, and males are affected three times more often than females. An organic cause is suspected, as the syndrome may follow physical disease of the brain, and many patients have minor neurological signs.

Haloperidol is an effective treatment. Behaviour therapy may also help.

Hypochondriasis (Kenyon, 1976)

Hypochondriasis can be an isolated symptom (primary hypochondriasis) or secondary to another psychiatric condition: obsessive-compulsive neurosis, a phobic anxiety state, hysterical neurosis, depression, or schizophrenia. The patient often fears a particular disease like cancer or VD, and in psychotic cases this fear may have delusional intensity. Dysmorphophobia is a related condition in which the patient believes that a part of his body looks abnormal.

Investigation to exclude genuine physical pathology is necessary, but should not be unduly extensive in case it encourages the patient to believe there is something physically wrong.

Pimozide may be effective in primary monosymptomatic hypochondriasis. In secondary cases, treatment depends on the underlying condition. Intractable severe cases may respond to leucotomy.

Insomnia (Berrios, 1980)

Insomnia, which is a very common complaint, may result from physical factors like pain, noise, stimulant drugs, or alcohol; from worry or unhappiness reactive to stress; or from psychiatric illness including anxiety neurosis, depressive illness, or dementia.

Complete sleep deprivation for more than 48 hours causes tiredness, lowered efficiency, and sometimes hallucinations. Partial sleep deprivation, although distressing, does not seem to have any serious consequences.

Insomnia is best treated by removing the cause. It is especially important to recognize depression when it presents with insomnia, as the correct treatment is an antidepressant not a hypnotic, and prescribing hypnotics may provide an easy means of suicide. If removal of the cause is impossible, hypnotics can be useful but should not be used for long periods as tolerance and dependence may develop. Hypnotics, also anti-depressants, reduce the proportion of REM sleep to orthodox sleep, with a rebound increase of REM sleep after they are discontinued; the significance of this is unknown.

Munchausen Syndrome (Reed, 1978)

Repeated simulation of illness resulting in hospital admission is termed the Munchausen syndrome, or hospital addiction syndrome. The patient, usually male, may undergo unpleasant investigations or treatment, but then discharge himself suddenly. Abdominal pain, chest pain, and vomiting or passing blood are common symptoms, but any physical or mental symptom may be described and patients may vary their complaints on different occasions. Many cases have a sociopathic personality, criminal tendencies, abuse drugs or alcohol, and are without fixed abode. It is difficult to study them in detail as they lie, use false names, and travel widely.

The condition may be a variety of hysteria, or may involve deliberate malingering. A masochistic desire to suffer, craving for attention, and antagonism towards the medical profession may be factors in the psycho-pathology. No treatment is known to be effective.

Paranoid States (Hamilton, 1978)

Paranoid states are characterized by ideas of reference, overvalued ideas or delusions, usually with a persecutory theme. They include:

1. *Acute paranoid reaction (bouffée délirante):* a transient state in which ideas of reference develop in response to stress.

2. *Paranoid personality development:* people of paranoid personality type become dominated by an overvalued idea.

3. *Paranoia:* a chronic condition in which there are fixed and elaborate delusions, without hallucinations, and with good preservation of the general personality.

4. *Paraphrenia:* as paranoia, with the addition of hallucinations.

5. *Paranoid schizophrenia:* delusions are prominent, but other features of schizophrenia are also present.

6. *Affective disorders:* paranoid delusions with or without hallucinations may occur in either the manic or depressed phases of affective psychoses.

7. *Organic states:* e.g. delirium from any cause, abuse of alcohol, amphetamines, or bromides.

Paranoid states are prone to develop in people who are isolated from others, whether because of living alone, being in a strange country with culture and language barriers, or being blind or deaf; and in those whose premorbid personality was of paranoid type. In psychodynamic terms, they can be explained by the mental mechanism of projection.

Folie à deux is the transfer of delusions, usually paranoid, from one person, the 'principal', to another, the 'associate'. The principal is psychotic, usually schizophrenic, and the associate may be psychotic also but is more often a person of dependent personality or low intelligence who has a close emotional involvement with the principal. If the pair are separated the associate usually gives up the delusions.

Very rarely there is more than one associate (*folie à trois, folie à quatre, folie à plusieurs*).

Morbid jealousy (Othello syndrome) (Shepherd, 1961) is an intense, groundless conviction that the subject's sexual partner is unfaithful. The underlying condition is a psychotic illness in about 40%, a neurosis or personality disorder in about 40%, alcoholism in about 5%, and organic brain disease in the rest. Men are affected twice as often as women. Sexual dysfunction is often present. Murder or suicide results in about 5% of cases. Treatment of the underlying condition or separation of the partners may be effective, but the condition tends to recur.

de Clérambault's syndrome (erotomania) is a delusion of being loved by another person, usually a stranger of higher social status. Women are affected more often than men, and most patients are without a real sexual partner. It may be secondary to another condition, usually schizophrenia, or be an isolated phenomenon. Treatment with phenothiazines may help to some extent.

Further Reading

The uncommon syndromes summarized in this chapter are described more fully in the book by Enoch and Trethowan (1979), and in the review article by Trethowan (1979).

References

Berrios, G. E. (1980). Sleep and its disorders. *Medicine*, **36**, 1875–1879.

Christodoulou, G. N. (1977). The syndrome of Capgras. *Br. J. Psychiatry*, **130**, 556–564.

Enoch, M. D., and Trethowan, W. H. (1979). *Uncommon Psychiatric Syndromes*. Wright, Bristol.

Hamilton, M. (1978). Paranoid states. *Br. J. Hosp. Med.*, **20**, 545–548.

Kenyon, F. E. (1976). Review article: hypochondriacal states. *Br. J. Psychiatry*, **129**, 1–14.

Parkes, C. M. (1965). Bereavement and mental illness. *Br. J. Med. Psychol.* **38**, 1–12 and 13–26.

Reed, J. L. (1978). Compensation neurosis and Munchausen syndrome. *Br. J. Hosp. Med.* **19**, 314–321.

Shepherd, M. (1961). Morbid jealousy. *J. Ment. Sci.*, **107**, 687–704.

Trethowan, W. H. (1979). Uncommon psychiatric disorders. *Br. J. Hosp. Med.* **22**, 490–495.

Whitty, C. W. M. (1978). Loss of memory as a clinical problem. *Br. J. Hosp. Med.*, **20**, 276–284.

CHAPTER 17

Psychiatry of Old Age

About 15% of the population are over 65, and this proportion is increasing. Psychiatric illness is more common among elderly people than in the general population, and the older they are the more common it is. This is probably because the elderly have a high prevalence of cerebral and systemic diseases which can cause organic brain syndromes, and because they are often subject to social and emotional stresses, e.g. death of the spouse, the loss of occupation, company and income which may follow retirement, deterioration in bodily functions, and the prospect of further aging and death.

Prevalence

Community surveys (Kay *et al.*, 1964) show the following approximate prevalence figures for psychiatric illness in those over 65:

Senile dementia	5% (15% over 75)
Other organic brain syndromes	5%
Functional psychoses	5%
Neuroses and personality disorders	10%

Clinical Features

Dementia and other organic brain syndromes are described in Chapter 7.

Depression (Jacoby, 1981) is the most common psychiatric illness in old people. First admission rates for depression are highest in the 50–70 age group.

Depression may be mistaken for dementia or simple aging, or be missed when it coexists with one of these. A trial of antidepressant treatment may be needed to resolve diagnostic uncertainty.

Depressive episodes usually recover with treatment, but the long-term prognosis is worse than for younger depressives in that about 70% develop future episodes.

108

Mania: first admission rates for mania show a slight increase with age. Transient depressive symptoms occur during the course of most manic illnesses in the elderly.

Physical illness or injuries easily result from self-neglect and over-activity, so that hospital treatment is desirable.

Schizophrenia (Kay, 1972): 14% of schizophrenic illnesses in women, and 4% in men, start after the age of 65, and almost always take the paranoid form with good preservation of the general personality.

Neuroses and personality disorders seldom start for the first time in old age, and an apparent first presentation at this time should raise suspicion of an underlying organic disorder or depressive illness.

Treatment

Psychotropic drugs should be used in small doses because in many old patients metabolism and excretion are inefficient, both therapeutic effects and side-effects are marked, and medical conditions necessitating caution in drug use are present. Compliance with drug treatment may be poor because of forgetfulness.

Barbiturates, benzodiazepines, and chlorpromazine are prone to cause severe side-effects and are best avoided. Suitable sedative drugs are chloral, chlormethiazole, promazine, thioridazine, and haloperidol.

ECT may be used if the patient is fit for anaesthetic.

Psychotherapy may be helpful although it will not achieve radical changes.

Psychiatric treatment should be accompanied by attention to physical health and social circumstances.

Organization of Services

Services are organized on the principle that most patients can be managed at home. Domiciliary visits are useful for deciding which cases require inpatient assessment or care.

Separate wards and day hospitals should be provided for elderly patients. The following provisions for a population of 200,000 are recommended (Department of Health and Social Security 1975):

1. 20 beds and 130 day places for functional illness;
2. 10–14 beds for assessment of organic confusional states;
3. 60–80 beds and 50–80 day places for long-term care of demented patients.

Admission wards discharge most of their patients home, or to alternative accommodation such as local authority warden-controlled housing or residential homes (Part 3), or privately run rest or nursing homes. Readmission at short notice should be available in crises. Temporary readmissions at planned intervals lessen the burden on families.

Care for patients outside hospital is given by the primary care team, community nurses, and the social services whose provisions include day centres, home helps, visiting, meals on wheels, and laundry.

Further Reading

Detailed accounts are provided by Isaacs and Post (1978) and Pitt (1974).

References

Department of Health and Social Security (1975). *Better Services for the Mentally Ill.* Cmnd. 6233. HMSO, London.

Isaacs, A. D., and Post, F. (1978). *Studies in Geriatric Psychiatry.* Wiley, Chichester.

Jacoby, R. J. (1981). Depression in the elderly. *Br. J. Hosp. Med.*, **25**, 40–47.

Kay, D. W. K. (1972). Schizophrenia and schizophrenia-like states in the elderly. *Br. J. Hosp. Med.*, **8**, 369–376.

Kay, D. W. K., Beamish, P., and Roth, M. (1964). Old age mental disorders in Newcastle-on-Tyne. Part 1: a study of prevalence. *Br. J. Psychiatry*, **110**, 146–158.

Pitt, B. (1974). Psychogeriatrics: *Introduction to the Psychiatry of Old Age.* Churchill Livingstone, Edinburgh.

CHAPTER 18

Child Psychiatry

Most psychiatric disorders of childhood involve a quantitative abnormality of emotion, conduct or rate of development. Emotions or conduct which are abnormal at one age may be normal at another.

Prevalence of Childhood Psychiatric Disorder

A community survey of 10–11 year olds on the Isle of Wight (Rutter *et al.*, 1970a,b) showed the prevalence of psychiatric disorder to be 7%: a similar survey of inner London found twice this prevalence, possibly due to a less favourable home or school environment (Rutter *et al.*, 1975b). Boys are affected twice as often as girls, and conduct disorders are twice as common as emotional disorders. During adolescence the rates increase, with more girls affected and a higher proportion of emotional disorders.

Only about 10% of children with psychiatric disorder are receiving psychiatric treatment.

Predisposing Factors

1. *Organic brain disorder* (associated with a 5-fold increase in rate).

2. *Non-neurological chronic physical disease* (associated with a 1.5-fold increase in rate).

3. *Low IQ*.

4. *Discord between the parents* or other family members, and undesirable parental attitudes including overprotection as well as hostility or neglect.

5. *Physical or mental illness* in another family member, especially the mother.

6. *Separation from the mother*, without an adequate substitute. Early work on maternal deprivation (Bowlby, 1951) suggested that it predisposed to 'affectionless psychopathy', antisocial behaviour, and retardation of mental and physical development. Later studies show that this is not necessarily so if the environment is otherwise good (Rutter, 1972).

7. *Adoption*.

8. *Illegitimacy*.

9. *Immigrant family*.

Classification

'Multi-axial' classification schemes such as the following have been proposed (Rutter *et al.*, 1975a):

First axis: clinical psychiatric syndrome
Psychoses.
Neurotic disorders, personality disorders and other non-psychotic mental disorders.
Adjustment reactions.
Disturbances of conduct not elsewhere classified.
Disturbance of emotions specific to childhood and adolescence.
Hyperkinetic syndrome of childhood.

Second axis: specific delays in development
Specific reading retardation.
Specific arithmetical retardation.
Other specific learning difficulties.
Developmental speech/language disorder.
Specific motor retardation.
Mixed developmental disorder.

Third axis: intellectual level

Fourth axis: associated medical conditions of aetiological importance

Fifth axis: associated abnormal psychosocial situations of aetiological importance

History-taking and Examination

The child and both parents need to be interviewed. Whether they are seen together or separately depends upon the age of the child and the preferences of those concerned. Most of this history has to be obtained from the parents, especially if the child is young. An interview with the parents may reveal problems of their own which are affecting the child, or have arisen through living with a disturbed child.

History:
1. Complaint.
2. History of present difficulties.
3. Family: age, occupation, mental and physical health of parents and siblings. A personal history of the parents including their own childhood. Emotional atmosphere of the household.
4. Developmental history:
   pregnancy—whether planned, medical complications.
   birth complications.
   milestones.
   illnesses.
5. School: academic achievements, social adjustment.
6. Life events.

Interview with child: children aged 8 or over can usually converse directly about their life and any problems in it. Information from younger children has to be obtained indirectly by observation of play or drawing, asking the child to invent stories or to give 'three wishes'.

Mental state: observation of mental state is carried out under the same headings used in adult psychiatry. Particular attention may be given to signs suggesting minor neurological impairment: over- or underactivity, poor coordination, short attention span.

Physical examination: this should include a neurological examination.

Psychological testing:
intelligence
educational achievements
personality assessment
motor and perceptual development.

Schoolteacher's report.

Social worker's report.

Treatment

Child Guidance Clinics are administered jointly by the Health, Education, and Social Services departments. They carry out multi-disciplinary treatment, the team being composed of child psychiatrist, educational psychologist, and social worker.

A psychotherapeutic approach is usually adopted. Individual psycho-therapy for the child enables him to express his anxieties to a trusted person, and receive encouragement in better methods of coping with difficulties. Sometimes a behavioural approach is appropriate. The parents are seen separately but concurrently by another therapist, usually a social worker. They may need to discuss their own problems, or may benefit from practical advice about dealing with the child. Family therapy may be given if the child's disturbance is thought to be secondary to a family disturbance.

Collaboration with other agencies may help, e.g. when the child has a physical disability or problems at school.

Psychotropic drugs are sometimes used in conjunction with these methods.

Relationship with Adult Disorder (Robins, 1966)

Children with conduct disorders, especially delinquency, often continue to behave antisocially in adult life.

Neurotic disorders in childhood, and the so-called 'neurotic traits' such as bed-wetting, nail-biting and stammering, are not associated with psychiatric disturbance in adult life.

Some individual conditions are described below.

DEVELOPMENTAL DISORDERS

Hyperkinetic Syndrome

The hyperkinetic syndrome is restlessness, inability to concentrate, and a short attention span.

Aggresive behaviour, mild mental handicap, epilepsy, minor motor abnormalities and minor EEG changes are sometimes associated with it. There is often a history of birth trauma, or other type of cerebral insult in early life, and so the syndrome is usually ascribed to 'minimal brain damage'.

The hyperkinetic syndrome is readily misdiagnosed, as many parents describe their children as abnormally overactive, and its existence has been questioned (Editorial, 1978). Differential diagnosis includes mania of early onset.

The most effective treatment is, paradoxically, a cerebral stimulant of the amphetamine group. Methylphenidate has been widely used. These drugs have many adverse effects including stunting growth. Primidone or phenothiazines may also help. Spontaneous improvement by adolescence is usual.

Speech and Language Disorders

Speech development may be delayed, abnormal, or absent because of deafness, mental handicap, sociocultural deprivation, developmental dysphasia, elective mutism (a form of negativistic behaviour usually occurring transiently in otherwise normal children), and autism.

Dyslexia (specific reading retardation)(Rutter and Yule, 1975) is an isolated difficulty in learning to read and write, occurring in children with no other handicaps.

These disabilities can often be improved by special teaching methods.

Enuresis (Kolvin *et al.*, 1973)

Urinary infection and other physical causes must always be excluded, although they are only present in a minority of cases.

Ninety per cent of 7 year olds are dry at night. Primary nocturnal enuresis is usually a result of delayed maturation rather than an indication of emotional disturbance. It often runs in families, and occasionally continues into adult life. Treatment includes lifting the child at night, a token economy regimen, and a buzzer and pad device. Tricyclic antidepressants are effective, probably due to their anticholinergic effects, but the use of such potentially toxic drugs for a benign condition should be avoided.

Secondary nocturnal enuresis is sometimes due to infection, more often to emotional disturbance. Both causes require specific treatment and should not be dealt with by the methods above.

Encopresis

Most 4 years olds are faecally continent. Physical causes e.g. Hirschsprung's disease, must be excluded.

Primary encopresis is usually the result of deficient training, and secondary encopresis a response to psychological stress.

Tics

A tic is a repetitive, purposeless movement, partly under voluntary control. Tics may develop in normal children, and are exacerbated by emotional disturbance. They are best ignored, and usually disappear spontaneously, but if not then behaviour therapy may help.

Gilles de la Tourette's syndrome (Chapter 16) often starts in childhood.

CONDUCT DISORDERS

Juvenile Delinquency (Scott, 1966)

Delinquency is law-breaking behaviour. Twenty per cent of teenage boys from large cities are convicted on one or more occasions, usually for stealing or destructiveness.

Subcultural influences are the most important cause. There is no genetic element but there is a strong association with disturbed home circumstances including family discord, criminality in other family members, and large families; it is also more common in certain areas of cities. Delinquency has a less marked association with brain damage, low intelligence, extraversion, and minor physical deformities.

About 40% of delinquent teenagers become criminals in adult life.

School Avoidance

Truanting is staying away from school to do something more enjoyable. Poor parental control, boredom at school, poor ability, and delinquent behaviour are associated with it.

School phobia is reluctance to attend school, either due to fear of teachers or other children, or more often to fear of separation from the mother. The mother often encourages it because she is reluctant to be separated from the child. The child may complain of headache or abdominal pain on school mornings. Treatment includes dealing with any contributory factors at school, psychotherapy for the child and mother, and encouragement to return to school as soon as possible (behaviour therapy may be helpful in this).

NEUROSES

Anxiety neurosis, obsessive–compulsive neurosis, and hysterical neurosis with conversion symptoms in their classical forms sometimes occur in childhood, but it is more usual for children to show diverse combinations of neurotic symptoms.

Isolated phobias and rituals are common in otherwise well adjusted children.

Depression in childhood is usually reactive to stress (Graham, 1974), often to a loss. Somatic symptoms, e.g. anorexia, abdominal pain, or headaches, are a frequent presentation. Suicide is very rare. Psychotherapy or tricyclic antidepressants may be effective. Bipolar affective disorder occasionally starts in childhood, with either depressive or manic episodes; manic ones may present as conduct disorders or hyperkinesis.

PSYCHOSES

'Childhood psychosis' includes:

1. *Disintegrative (or developmental) psychosis:* a child aged 2 or 3 becomes emotionally withdrawn, loses speech, deteriorates intellectually, and shows emotional and behavioural disturbances.

Schilder's disease, lipoidoses, and degenerative changes of obscure aetiology are among the causes of this rare condition.

2. *Schizophrenia* occasionally starts in childhood.

3. *Autism.*

Autism (Kanner's Syndrome) (Wing, 1970)

Kanner (1943) described autism as a syndrome of withdrawal from people, and language abnormalities. It is now believed to be an organic disorder. Theories that it is a form of schizophrenia, precipitated by abnormal parental attitudes, are now discredited.

The prevalence of autism is 4.5 per 10,000 children, and it is more common in boys.

Seventy per cent of patients are mentally handicapped, often due to a specific cause such as rubella, while their parents' intelligence is often above average. Twin studies suggest that there is a genetic predisposition. Twenty-five per cent have neurological impairments and 30% develop epilepsy during adolescence.

Symptoms start within the first 3 years of life and include abnormal response to sound, failure to understand speech, and either mutism or abnormal forms of speech such as echolalia, nominal aphasia, and pronoun reversal, aloofness from people, and insistence on rituals and routines.

Autistic children have a bad prognosis and often need institutional care. The lower the IQ the worse the prognosis is. Special education may improve the language disorder.

PSYCHOSOMATIC DISORDERS

Eating Disorders

Anorexia is usually the result of physical ill-health. Excessive parental concern about food can result in anorexia, or lead the child to manipulate the parents by refusing to eat or by vomiting. Depression is another cause. Anorexia nervosa occasionally occurs in prepubertal children.

Overeating is often a compensation for emotional deprivation. In adolescence, overeating usually causes obesity (and hence further emotional difficulties), but this is not always so in younger children, who may remain undersized (deprivational dwarfism).

Pica is eating the inedible. Exploration of objects with the mouth is normal from 6 to 12 months of age, but may continue for years in blind or mentally handicapped children. Sucking lead-painted objects may cause mental handicap.

Periodic Syndrome

The periodic syndrome consists of a cluster of some or all of five symptoms, which recur at intervals: vomiting, headache, abdominal pain, limb pain, and fever. It affects anxious children under stress. They often develop migraine in later life.

Physical diseases in children which are believed to have a psychosomatic element include asthma, eczema, and ulcerative colitis.

NON-ACCIDENTAL INJURY TO CHILDREN (Scott, 1977)

Non-accidental injury to children, or baby battering, is known to cause at least 150 deaths and 8000 cases of injury annually in England and Wales.

Parents who injure their children are typically young, immature, poor, and have disturbed home backgrounds themselves. A small minority are mentally ill. There is a raised incidence of factors likely to impair 'bonding' between parents and child: unwanted pregnancy, complications during pregnancy or birth, separations between parents and child, and ill-health in the child.

Bony injuries, including fractures and periosteal haemorrhage, and soft tissue damage like bruises, retinal haemorrhage and cigarette burns, are common. The child is usually retarded in both mental and physical development.

Social Services departments are responsible for prevention and management, and keep a register of children at risk, although the value of doing so is unknown. A conference about any suspected or confirmed case is held, attended by social services and any other professionals involved: police, health visitor, GP, psychiatrist. It may be necessary for battered children to be taken into care, but if the parents are anxious to keep the child at home and change their behaviour, provision of appropriate help and close surveillance may succeed.

PSYCHIATRY OF ADOLESCENCE (Wolkind and Coleman, 1976)

10–20% of those aged 12–18 have psychiatric disorders. These include:

1. *'Adolescent turmoil':* problems stem from the processes involved in developing an individual personality, such as acquiring independence from the parents, sexual maturation, and making social relationships. This may cause anxiety or depression, rebellion against parents and authorities, and experimentation with contrasting behaviours. Extreme forms are termed 'identity crises'.

2. *Persisting childhood disorders.*

3. *Onset of adult disorders:* schizophrenia, affective disorders, and neuroses may all begin during adolescence. Personality disorders may first become evident under the stress of growing up, but the personality may mature later and so a firm diagnosis cannot be made at this age.

4. *Drug or alcohol abuse.*

Diagnosis may require prolonged observation as it may be difficult to distinguish severe 'adolescent turmoil' from psychiatric illness. Treatment of seriously disturbed adolescents may be carried out in a residential adolescent unit. Such units usually keep patients for several months and use psychotherapeutic treatment which may or may not include the patient's family. The DHSS recommends 25 beds per 100,000 population for psychiatrically disturbed adolescents.

Further Reading

A detailed account of child psychiatry is given by Rutter and Hersov (1977), and a shorter one by Barker (1979).

References

Barker, P. (1979). *Basic Child Psychiatry.* Crosby Lockwood Staples, London.

Bowlby, J. (1951). *Maternal Care and Mental Health.* WHO Monograph Series, No. 2, Geneva.

Editorial (1978). Hyperactivity. *Lancet,* **2**, 561.

Graham, P. J. (1974). Depression in pre-pubertal children. *Dev. Med. Child. Neurol.,* **16**, 340–349.

Kanner, L. (1943). Autistic disturbances of affective contact. *Nerv. Child.,* **2**, 217–250.

Kolvin, I., MacKeith, R., and Meadow, S. R. (Eds.) (1973). *Bladder Control and Enuresis.* Clinics in Devel. Med., Nos. 48/49. SIMP/Heinemann, London.

Robins, L. (1966). *Deviant Children Grown Up.* Williams and Wilkins, Baltimore.

Rutter, M. L. (1972). *Maternal Deprivation Reassessed.* Penguin, Harmondsworth.

Rutter, M. L., Graham, P. J., and Yule, W. (1970a). *A Neuropsychiatric Study in Childhood.* Clinics in Devel. Med., Nos. 35/36. SIMP/Heinemann, London.

Rutter, M. L., and Hersov, L. (Eds.) (1977). *Child Psychiatry: Modern Approaches.* Blackwell Scientific Publications, Oxford.

Rutter, M. L., Shaffer, D., and Shepherd, M. (1975a). *A Multiaxial Classification of Child Psychiatric Disorders.* WHO, Geneva.

Rutter, M. L., Tizard, J., and Whitmore, K. (Eds.) (1970b). *Education, Health and Behaviour.* Longman, London.

Rutter, M. L., and Yule, W. (1975). The concept of specific reading retardation. *J. Child. Psychol. Psychiatry,* **16**, 181–197.

Rutter, M. L., Yule, B., Quinton, D., Rowlands, O., Yule, W., and Berger, M. (1975b). Attainment and adjustment in two geographic areas: III. Some factors accounting for area differences. *Br. J. Psychiatry,* **126**, 520–533.

Scott, P. D. (1966). Medical aspects of delinquency. *Br. J. Hosp. Med.,* **1**, 219–223 and 259.

Scott, P. D. (1977). Non-accidental injury in children. *Br. J. Psychiatry*, **131**, 366–380.

Wing, L. (1970). The syndrome of early childhood autism. *Br. J. Hosp. Med.*, **4**, 381–392.

Wolkind, S. N. and Coleman, J. C. (1976). The psychiatry of adolescence. *Br. J. Hosp. Med.*, **15**, 575–582.

CHAPTER 19

Mental Handicap

Definition

The Mental Health Act 1959 (using the alternative term 'sub-normality') gives the following definitions:

Subnormality: a state of arrested or incomplete development of mind which includes subnormality of intelligence and is of a nature or degree which requires or is susceptible to medical treatment, or other special care or training.

Severe subnormality: a state of arrested or incomplete development of mind which includes subnormality of intelligence and is of a nature or degree that the patient is incapable of living an independent life or of guarding himself against serious exploitation, or will be so incapable when of an age to do so.

IQ levels are about 50–69 for 'subnormality' and below 49 for 'severe subnormality'. The definitions, however, depend upon the presence of social incompetence, which is determined by factors other than IQ.

Terminology

'Mental handicap', 'mental subnormality', 'mental defect', and 'mental retardation' are alternative terms.

The terms formerly used to designate the various degrees of handicap include:

IQ 50–69	High-grade subnormal
	Mildly retarded
	ESN
	Feeble-minded
	Moron
IQ 20–49	Medium-grade subnormal

	Retarded
	Imbecile
IQ 0–19	Low-grade subnormal
	Profoundly retarded
	Idiot

Prevalence

In the general population, 2.5% have an IQ below 70, and 0.4% below 50. Most people with an IQ between 50 and 70, however, are competent to live in the community and do not need special facilities.

Causes

About 70% of mild cases do not have one isolated cause, but belong to the so-called 'subcultural' group, in which the handicap results from the combination of a poor genetic intellectual endowment and an upbringing which is either educationally or emotionally deprived. Mild handicap correlates with low social class, poverty, overcrowding, large family size, and family disruption. The other 30% of mild cases have brain damage.

Most severe cases are associated with a specific organic pathology. About 35% have a genetic or chromosomal abnormality (Down's syndrome being the most frequent), and about 65% have acquired brain damage.

The specific causes can be classified as follows:

1. *Chromosomal or genetic abnormalities*, e.g. Down's syndrome, phenylketonuria.

2. *Primary maldevelopments of the brain of obscure aetiology*, e.g. spina bifida with hydrocephalus, microgyria.

3. *Prenatal damage by factors affecting the mother*, e.g. rubella, cytomegalovirus, toxoplasmosis, syphilis, irradiation, malnutrition, alcoholism, teratogenic drugs.

4. *Perinatal damage*, e.g. birth trauma, anoxia, Rhesus incompatibility.

5. *Postnatal damage*, e.g. encephalitis, lead poisoning, head injury.

Investigation of the cause involves a personal history, family history, physical examination, chromosome studies, and testing blood and urine for abnormal metabolites.

If a cause is discovered there may be an appropriate treatment, e.g. special diets for certain enzyme defects, and it enables genetic counselling to be given to the patient's relatives.

Some of the specific causes are described in more detail below.

Diagnosis

Severe cases are usually obvious from infancy, because they have behavioural defects, and frequently physical abnormalities too. Mild cases are less obvious, but affected children develop more slowly than normal, and are found to have low scores on routine IQ testing. A detailed psychological, medical, and social assessment is required to determine the degree of handicap, and to enable decisions about aims and methods of management.

Differential diagnosis includes deafness and emotional disturbance.

Associated Phenomena

1. *Physical defects* are present in about a third of severe cases.

2. *Epilepsy* is present in about 25%, being more frequent the lower the IQ. The same lesion is usually responsible for both the fits and the low IQ.

3. *Psychiatric illness* (Snaith and James, 1979) is present in about 10%. Patients seldom have the linguistic ability to describe psychiatric symptoms, and so may present only with behaviour disturbance, which makes diagnosis difficult.

4. *Behaviour disturbance* is present in about half the severely handicapped, and patients' families often request their admission to hospital on this account. Its causes include:

   (a) a direct manifestation of the underlying brain damage.
   (b) psychiatric illness.
   (c) frustration with a boring or repressive environment.
   (d) excessive or inappropriate medication.

Behaviour disturbance may be considered to include the absence of desirable behaviour of which the patient is potentially capable, e.g. speech or self-care, as well as the presence of undesirable behaviour, e.g. aggressiveness, overactivity or self-mutilation.

Treatment

Multidisciplinary management has found useful application with the mentally handicapped.

The medical contribution includes diagnosis and treatment of both physical and psychiatric problems. Drugs and other physical methods of treatment are sometimes indicated, but the excessive use of tranquillizers and anticonvulsants must be avoided. These drugs may exacerbate intellectual impairment besides having other side-effects. Measurement of blood anti-convulsant levels should be done to help find the optimum dose.

Psychologists are involved in assessing patients' overall intelligence, and any specific defects or abilities. They also plan behavioural treatment methods, usually those derived from operant conditioning theory, which can be useful even in the severely handicapped for teaching self-care, practical skills, and improving social behaviour. Desirable behaviour or the acquisition of skills is given positive reinforcement by a tangible reward or approving attention. Undesirable behaviour may be a means of seeking attention, in which case it may be best ignored; alternatively it can be managed by occupying patients with more productive activities instead, or removing them to a 'time-out' room for a few minutes as soon as it begins. Token economy regimens, in which a whole ward is run on these lines, can be used for patients capable of understanding them.

Social and educational aspects of treatment are important. An improved environment has been shown to raise IQ levels of children with 'subcultural' handicap. Patients may live at home, in sheltered accommodation such as community home or hostel provided by the local authority, or in hospital. Hospital care is now discouraged except for the very severely handicapped (Department of Health and Social Security, 1971). Eighty per cent of severely handicapped children, and 20% of adults, live with their families. Most parents prefer to keep a mentally handicapped child at home, although those who do so have an increased liability to social and financial problems. Such problems could be lessened by better community services.

The mildly handicapped are placed in ordinary schools if possible. Special schools, ESN(M) and ESN(S), exist for the others. Further training after school-leaving age is provided in adult training centres and social education centres. Some patients can hold jobs in the community, and others are employed in sheltered workshops.

Prognosis

Mild cases have a good prognosis in that they usually become capable of living independently. They sometimes develop late and achieve an IQ within the normal range by the time they reach adult life.

Severe cases need permanent care, and have a reduced life expectancy.

Prevention

Up to half the number of cases of mental handicap could probably be prevented by application of the following methods:

1. *Improved antenatal and obstetric care*, e.g. rubella immunization for girls, treatment of Rhesus incompatibility, special care of low birth weight babies.

2. *Improved infant welfare*, e.g. immunization programmes, early detection of mild mental handicap and of impaired sight and hearing.

3. *Screening of neonates*, e.g. routine urine testing to detect phenyl-ketonuria.

4. *Genetic counselling*, e.g. calculating the precise risk of handicap in future children of those parents who have an existing child handicapped by a genetic or chromosomal abnormality; and detection of the carrier state in relatives of those with a recessive condition.

5. *Amniocentesis:* amniotic fluid is sampled at 16 weeks gestation, and fetal fibroblasts examined for chromosomal or genetic abnormalities. The indications are:

(a) raised alpha-feto protein level in maternal blood, causes of which include open spina bifida.
(b) congenital abnormalities in previous babies.
(c) mothers over 35 years old, who have an increased risk of having babies with Down's syndrome.

Amniocentesis carries a small risk of causing abortion, antepartum haemorrhage, and orthopaedic deformities.

There is no point in performing amniocentesis unless the mother wants an abortion if fetal abnormality is detected.

A complete screening for all detectable biochemical abnormalities is not practicable, so it is necessary to know which one requires exclusion. The conditions which can be diagnosed by amniocentesis include:

(a) chromosome abnormalities.

(b) open spina bifida.

(c) certain biochemical abnormalities including the mucopolysaccharidoses, Lesch–Nyhan syndrome, and Tay–Sach's disease.

Conditions for which no test is yet available include Huntington's chorea and tuberose sclerosis.

Some of the specific causes of mental handicap will be described.

GENETIC CAUSES

Autosomal Chromosome Abnormalities

Down's syndrome (mongolism) (Scully, 1973) is caused by one of two abnormalities, trisomy 21 or translocation of chromosome 21.

Trisomy 21 becomes more frequent with increasing maternal age:

Maternal age	Frequency of trisomy 21 per 1000 births
under 35	1
35–39	4
40–44	13
over 45	35

Trisomy 21 does not run in families.

Translocation of chromosome 21 is not related to maternal age. It may result from mosaicism in either parent, in which case there is a likelihood of recurrence of Down's syndrome in future pregnancies, or it may occur sporadically.

Down's syndrome is the commonest specific cause of mental handicap, occurring in 1 per 650 live births.

Mental handicap is inevitable, and usually severe. Other features are a friendly temperament, a typical facial appearance with slanting palpebral fissures, a short little finger with only one palmar crease ('trident hand' and 'simian crease'), hypotonic muscles, cardiac defects (in 10% of patients), and a high susceptibility to chest infections, lymphatic leukaemia, and premature aging. Most patients die by early adult life.

Less common chromosome abnormalities include trisomy D (Pateau's syndrome), trisomy E (Edward's syndrome), and the *'cri du chat'* syndrome.

Sex Chromosome Abnormalities

Sex chromosome abnormalities are described here although they are not always associated with mental handicap.

Male phenotype

The XYY syndrome (Pitcher, 1971) is found in about 21 per 1000 men in high security hospitals, as opposed to 1.5 per 1000 men in the general population, and so is presumed to predispose to criminal behaviour. Other abnormalities sometimes associated with it include low IQ, infertility, neurological disorders, skeletal disorders, and myopia. Some cases are phenotypically normal.

The XXY syndrome (Klinefelter's syndrome) comprises hypogonadism, infertility, an effeminate appearance, and usually low IQ. Neurotic symptoms are frequent, probably because of the stigma of the other abnormalities.

Female phenotype

The XO syndrome (Turner's syndrome) comprises ovarian dysgenesis, short stature, a webbed neck, and sometimes cardiac malformations. IQ is normal. There may be a raised susceptibility to anorexia nervosa.

The XXX syndrome (superfemale) is associated with low IQ, but appearance and fertility are normal. Women with more than three X chromosomes exist, and are mentally handicapped with numerous physical abnormalities.

Autosomal Dominant Gene Abnormalities

Tuberose sclerosis (epiloia) is characterized by severe mental handicap, epilepsy, and adenoma sebaceum. Nodules of neuroglia, sometimes calcified, occur in the brain, and show on brain scan. Muscular and vascular tumours occur in various organs. Adenoma sebaceum is a nodular malformation on the cheeks which has vascular and sebaceous components and appears after a few years of life. *'Café au lait* spots' and 'shagreen patches' occur on the skin. Partial versions of the syndrome occur, probably due to incomplete penetrance of the gene.

Autosomal Recessive Gene Abnormalities

Phenylketonuria occurs in 4 per 100,000 live births, and usually results from a defect in phenylalanine hydroxylase, the enzyme which converts phenylalanine to tyrosine. A few cases result from other defects in the subsequent metabolic pathway. Phenylpyruvic acid and other abnormal metabolites of phenylalanine are present in the urine after 3 weeks of age, enabling a screening test to be carried out. Carriers of the gene can be detected by a phenylalanine loading test, for genetic counselling purposes.

Patients have fair colouring, because melanin production is impaired.

Untreated cases have severe mental handicap, but if a low phenyl-alanine diet is started in infancy and continued until the age of 10, intellectual development may approach normal.

Other aminoacidurias include homocystinuria (in which there may be schizophreniform symptoms), Hartnup disease, and maple syrup urine disease.

Galactosaemia results from a defect of T galactose uridyltransferase, the enzyme which converts galactose to glucose. Vomiting, jaundice, and hepatosplenomegaly are present from infancy, and cataracts develop later. It can be detected by the finding of galactose in the urine. A diet free from milk and other galactose-containing foods ameliorates the symptoms.

Tay–Sach's disease is a degenerative condition of the central nervous system due to an abnormality of lipid metabolism. A cherry-red spot appears on the macula after a few months of age, and is followed by optic atrophy and blindness. Fits usually occur. The disease leads to death at about the age of 2. Its prevalence is highest in Jews.

Hurler's syndrome (gargoylism) is a disorder of mucopolysaccharides, which accumulate in the brain, and in other organs with consequent hepatosplenomegaly. Most patients have an aggressive temperament.

Hunter's syndrome (which has sex-linked recessive inheritance) and *Sanfilipino's syndrome* are similar.

Gaucher's, Niemann–Pick's and Hand–Schüller–Christian diseases are all lipid storage diseases, which are most common in Jews.

Laurence–Moon–Biedl syndrome comprises mental handicap, retinitis pigmentosa, polydactyly, obesity, and hypogonadism. Partial versions occur.

Microcephaly comprises severe mental handicap, overactivity, and a low cephalic index which gives a bird-like appearance. The term 'microcephaly' is also used for the mental handicap with reduced cephalic size which may result from other causes, e.g. radiation or cytomegalovirus infection in intrauterine life.

Hypothyroidism due to deficiency of one of the enzymes involved in thyroid hormone synthesis causes general retardation of development with lethargy and a puffy appearance. Symptoms are ameliorated by lifelong thyroxine replacement therapy.

Sex-linked Recessive

Lesch–Nyhan syndrome results from accumulation of uric acid due to a defect of purine metabolism. There is severe handicap, self-mutilation, spasticity and choreoathetosis.

ACQUIRED CAUSES

Prenatal Infections

Cytomegalovirus is the commonest form of intrauterine infection to cause mental handicap. The mother is usually symptom-free. The child has microcephaly, necrotizing haemorrhagic encephalitis and intracerebral calcification. 50% die soon after birth. A vaccine against cytomegalovirus is currently being developed.

Congenital syphilis causes mental handicap, deafness, keratitis, and malformation of the teeth, and GPI develops in adolescence. Serological tests may be negative. It can be prevented by serological testing on pregnant women with antisyphilitic treatment for them if required.

Toxoplasmosis is a protozoal infection which causes mental handicap, choroidoretinitis, and miliary intracranial calcification. Maternal infection can be detected by serological testing.

Maternal rubella is only likely to harm the fetus during the first trimester. It causes mental handicap, deafness, cataract, and cardiac lesions.

Birth Complications

Birth injury may cause hemiplegia, paraplegia, or quadriplegia, usually associated with mental handicap, and often with epilepsy.

Rhesus incompatibility, if severe enough to cause kernicterus, is likely to result in extrapyramidal rigidity, athetosis, and mental handicap.

Post-natal Damage

Lead poisoning may result from sucking lead-painted objects, or exposure to high concentrations of petrol fumes. It causes mild mental handicap, anaemia with basophil stippling of red cells, and a 'lead line' on the gums and epiphyses. The importance of mild degrees of lead poisoning is uncertain.

Other Causes

Hydrocephalus has several possible causes: the congenital malformation of the fourth ventricle which may be associated with spina bifida, meningitis, or a brain stem tumour in childhood, or rarely a sex-linked inherited condition. Insertion of a shunt ameliorates brain damage.

Further Reading

A short account of mental handicap is given by Heaton-Ward (1975); longer ones by Kirman and Bicknell (1975) and Clarke and Clarke (1974).

References

Clarke, A. M. and Clarke, A. D. B. (Eds.) (1974). *Mental Deficiency. The Changing Outlook*. Methuen, London.
Department of Health and Social Security (1971). *Better Services for the Mentally Handicapped*. HMSO, London.

Heaton-Ward, W. A. (1975). *Mental Subnormality.* Wright, Bristol.

Kirman, B., and Bicknell, J. (1975). *Mental Handicap.* Churchill Livingstone, Edinburgh.

Pitcher, D. (1971). The XYY syndrome. *Br. J. Hosp. Med.* **5**, 379–393.

Scully, C. (1973). Down's syndrome. *Br. J. Hosp. Med.*, **10**, 89–98.

Snaith, R. P. and James, F. E. (Eds.) (1979). *Psychiatric Illness and Mental Handicap.* Gaskell, London.

CHAPTER 20

Psychopharmacology

Some obvious questions which are often forgotten when psychotropic drugs are used include the following.

1. Are the symptoms likely to respond to drugs at all? Antidepressants, for example, are unlikely to help unhappiness secondary to social problems.
2. If a drug does not appear to work, has it been given in adequate dosage for a long enough time? Depressive illness treated with antidepressants, and schizophrenia treated with neuroleptics, may take three or four weeks to respond.
3. Do the therapeutic effects outweigh any unwanted ones? Side-effects, allergic or idiosyncratic reactions may affect any body system; tolerance or dependence may develop; the drug may interact with other drugs or with alcohol. There is an increased danger of side-effects in patients who are elderly or physically ill. Psychotropic drugs should only be used in women who are pregnant or breast-feeding if they are essential, although there is no evidence that those in current use cause serious damage to the baby.
4. Is the patient taking the drug as prescribed? About a third of patients given psychotropic drugs do not taken them, whereas others take them in excess. Psychotropic drugs are the commonest means of deliberate self-poisoning, and large quantities should not be prescribed to patients with suicidal tendencies.
5. Is the drug still necessary? Minor tranquillizers for anxiety or insomnia should preferably be used for only a few weeks at a time. A course of antidepressants should last several months. Lithium for prophylaxis of affective disorder, and neuroleptics for maintenance treatment of schizophrenia, are usually continued for several years but may not be required indefinitely, or may have to be stopped if serious long-term side-effects develop.

The main groups of psychotropic drugs in use today are described below.

NEUROLEPTICS (Table 1)

Neuroleptics, or major tranquillizers, have ameliorating effects on psychotic symptoms, as well as a general sedative action.

They include phenothiazines, thioxanthenes, butyrophenones, and diphenylbutylpiperidines.

Table 1 Neuroleptics

Phenothiazines

Chlorpromazine (Largactil)	Promazine (Sparine)
Fluphenazine (Modecate)	Thiopropazate (Dartalan)
Methotrimeprazine (Veractil)	Thioproperazine (Majeptil)
Pericyazine (Neulactil)	Thioridazine (Melleril)
Perphenazine (Fentazin)	Trifluoperazine (Stelazine)
Prochlorperazine (Stemetil)	

Thioxanthenes

Chlorprothixene (Taractan)	Flupenthixol (Depixol)
Clopenthixol (Clopixol)	Thiothixene (Navane)

Butyrophenones

Benperidol (Anquil)	Haloperidol (Haldol, Serenace)
Droperidol (Droleptan)	Trifluperidol (Triperidol)

Diphenylbutylpiperidines

Fluspirilene (Redeptin)	Pimozide (Orap)

Indications
1. Schizophrenia.
2. Mania.
3. Acute disturbance from other causes.
4. Anxiety which has failed to respond to 'minor' tranquillizers.
5. In general medicine as antiemetics and to potentiate analgesics and anaesthetics.

Pharmacology

Neuroleptics block dopamine receptors in the mesolimbic area, and this is probably the mechanism of their antipsychotic effect. Increase of serum prolactin is a measure of dopaminergic blockade.

Most of them also block cerebral receptors for noradrenaline, and periphally they have antiadrenergic, anticholinergic, and antihistaminic actions.

Administration

Control of an acute psychosis is achieved by giving a neuroleptic in divided doses, three or four times daily. There is a calming effect from the start, but full response may take three or four weeks. The drug is usually given as tablets or syrup, but intramuscular injections can be used if rapid sedation is required. Chlorpromazine is the usual drug of first choice for schizophrenia, and haloperidol for mania.

Long-term neuroleptic treatment of schizophrenia is often given by slow-release intramuscular injections of fluphenazine decanoate, flupenthixol decanoate, clopenthixol decanoate, or fluspirilene, every 1–4 weeks. Such injections are superior for some patients in whom oral preparations are incompletely absorbed or undergo rapid first-pass metabolism in the liver, but their main advantage is that their use ensures regular medication and follow-up.

Side-effects

1. *Neurological and psychiatric:* drowsiness, depression, fits, and akinesia may occur, but the commonest side-effects are extrapyramidal ones. *Parkinsonism* with tremor, rigidity, bradykinesia, and sialorrhoea may develop a few days or weeks after starting a neuroleptic, and is very frequent with high doses. *Akathisia*, mental agitation combined with motor restlessness, may develop over a similar period. A less frequent extrapyramidal effect is acute *dystonia*, including torticollis, other abnormal postures, and oculogyric crisis, soon after the drug is started. Extrapyramidal side-effects respond to anticholinergic antiparkinsonian drugs, but these drugs should not be given unless required because they may produce side-effects themselves.

Tardive dyskinesia is an extrapyramidal syndrome which may develop after neuroleptics have been given for more than a few months. Patients who are middle aged or elderly, female, or brain damaged are most likely to be affected. Antiparkinsonian drugs may encourage its development. Involuntary movements of choreiform or athetoid type affect the orofacial muscles and sometimes also the limbs or trunk. The cause may be proliferation or hypersensitivity of dopamine receptors after prolonged blockade by neuroleptics, or an imbalance between dopamine and its antagonists acetylcholine and GABA. Many drugs have been tried for the treatment of tardive dyskinesia (Mackay and Sheppard, 1979) including dopamine receptor blockers (thiopropazate, haloperidol, pimozide, metoclopramide, tiapride) which may produce temporary improvement but eventually make the dyskinesia worse; dopamine depleting drugs (tetrabenazine, reserpine, oxypertine, alpha methyldopa); dopamine-potentiating drugs (apomorphine, amantidine, methylphenidate, L-dopa, bromocriptine); cholinergic drugs (physostigmine, deanol, choline, lecithin); and GABA-potentiating drugs (baclofen, sodium valproate, benzodiazepines). Some cases of tardive dyskinesia do not respond to any of these treatments, and so it is desirable to prevent the development of the condition by keeping the dose of neuroleptics to a minimum, and using antiparkinsonian drugs with them only if necessary. Stopping neuroleptics for a few weeks each year (drug holidays) is probably not an effective method of preventing tardive dyskinesia.

2. *Cardiovascular:* hypotension, cardiac arrhythmias, oedema.

3. *Gastrointestinal:* dry mouth or excess salivation, constipation.

4. *Endocrine and metabolic:* weight gain, galactorrhoea, amenorrhoea, reduced fertility, false positive pregnancy tests.

5. *Haematological:* bone marrow depression.

6. *Ocular:* blurred vision, glaucoma, retinal pigmentation causing blindness, lens opacities.

7. *Genitourinary:* retention of urine, polyuria, impotence.

8. *Allergic:* cholestatic jaundice, rash, photosensitivity.

9. *Other:* sweating, nasal congestion.

Contraindications

Liver damage.

Tolerance and Dependence

These do not occur.

Metabolism

Phenothiazines are metabolized in the liver. Several hundred metabolites have been identified, some of which have neuroleptic activity and persist in the body for months.

Drug Interactions

Opiates, barbiturates, alcohol, other cerebral depressants, tricyclic antidepressants, and anticholinergic drugs are potentiated. Amphetamines are blocked.

Choice of Drug

The many phenothiazines available differ slightly from each other in side-effects and potency. Chlorpromazine was the first to be introduced and remains the most widely used. Trifluoperazine is less sedative, and probably more effective for treating delusions, but more likely to cause Parkinsonism. Thioridazine is less prone to cause Parkinsonism, but more prone to cause both tardive dyskinesia and retinal pigmentation. Promazine is milder, and suitable for the elderly.

A patient who has failed to respond to one phenothiazine is unlikely to respond to another, and should be given a butyrophenone or thioxanthene.

Butyrophenones cause prominent extrapyramidal side-effects, but fewer autonomic side-effects than phenothiazines.

TRICYLIC ANTIDEPRESSANTS (Table 2)

Imipramine and amitriptyline are the longest established drugs of this group. Many newer ones exist. Some newer antidepressants have a tetracyclic or other structure instead of a tricyclic one.

Indications

1. Depressive illness.
2. Depression occurring in association with other psychiatric conditions.
3. Nocturnal enuresis.

Pharmacology

The likely mechanism of antidepressant action is prevention of reuptake of amine neurotransmitters into neurones. Some of the

Table 2 Antidepressant drugs

Tricyclics
Amitriptyline (Tryptizol, Lentizol)
Butriptyline (Evadyne)
Clomipramine (Anafranil)
Desipramine (Pertofran)
Dibenzepin (Noveril)
Dothiepin (Prothiaden)
Doxepin (Sinequan)
Imipramine (Tofranil)
Iprindole (Prondol)
Nortriptyline (Allegron, Aventyl)
Protriptyline (Concordin)
Trimipramine (Surmontil)
Tetracyclics
Maprotiline (Ludiomil)
Mianserin (Bolvidon, Norval)
Other new antidepressants
Nomifensine (Merital)
Trazodone (Molipaxin)
Viloxazine (Vivalan)
MAOIs
Isocarboxazid (Marplan)
Phenelzine (Nardil)
Tranylcypromine (Parnate)

drugs prevent reuptake of 5HT, others that of noradrenaline. Most of these drugs have peripheral anticholinergic effects.

Administration

Tricyclics need to be given for up to three weeks before their anti-depressant effect is manifest, and should be continued several months after apparent recovery. They should be started in a small dose, which can be increased in a few days if side-effects such as drowsiness, dry mouth, or postural hypotension are not troublesome. They are usually given orally; injectable preparations exist but have no proven advantage. Those drugs with sedative properties may be given in a single dose at night to help sleep, minimize side-effects during the day, and simplify administration.

Drugs of tertiary tricyclic structure (amitriptyline, imipramine, trimipramine, clomipramine) should be given in the largest dose which the patient can tolerate, since their therapeutic effect increases with their plasma concentration. Drugs of secondary tricyclic structure (nortriptyline, desipramine, protriptyline) are most effective in the middle range of plasma concentration, so that it is impossible to judge the optimum dose unless concentrations are measured.

Side-Effects

1. *Neurological and psychiatric:* confusion, excitement, mania in predisposed subjects, drowsiness, sleep disturbance, nightmares, hallucinations, headaches, fits, ataxia, extrapyramidal symptoms, peripheral neuropathy, exacerbation of schizophrenic symptoms.

2. *Cardiovascular:* postural hypotension, tachycardia, prolonged QT interval and other ECG changes, cardiac arrhythmias, heart block, precipitation of myocardial infarction or strokes.

3. *Gastrointestinal:* dry mouth, black tongue, nausea, constipation, occasionally paralytic ileus.

4. *Endocrine and metabolic:* weight gain, galactorrhoea, gynaecomastia, testicular swelling, blood sugar change.

5. *Haematological:* bone marrow depression, eosinophilia, purpura.

6. *Ocular:* blurred vision, precipitation of glaucoma.

7. *Genitourinary:* retention of urine.

8. *Allergic:* rash, urticaria, oedema.

9. *Other:* sweating, jaundice.

Contraindications

Cardiac disease, glaucoma, and prostatic enlargement may be absolute or relative contraindications depending on their severity in relation to the severity of the depression.

Tolerance and Dependence

If treatment is stopped suddenly there can be a withdrawal syndrome of nausea, headache, sweating, and insomnia.

Drug Interactions

Tricyclics potentiate monoamine oxidase inhibitors, barbiturates, phenothiazines, alcohol, anticoagulants, anticholinergics, and local anaesthetics.

They decrease the efficacy of some hypotensives: bethanidine, guanethidine, debrisoquine, clonidine, reserpine.

Choice of Drug

If one antidepressant drug fails, another one may succeed. In future, biochemical tests to identify the most effective drugs for an individual patient may become available. There is some evidence that patients with low urinary levels of MHPG (methoxy-hydroxy-phenylethylene glycol) which is a metabolite of noradrenaline, respond to imipramine, whereas those with high levels respond to amitriptyline.

Patients with agitated depression are usually given one of the more sedative drugs of the group, e.g. amitriptyline, dothiepin, doxepin, trimipramine, maprotiline, mianserin, whereas retarded patients are given one which is neutral or stimulant, e.g. imipramine, nortriptyline, nomifensine.

Side-effects may determine the choice of drug. The newer compounds do not appear to be any more effective as antidepressants than the older ones, but do have less marked side-effects and are safer in overdose. Mianserin, iprindole, nomifensine, and trazodone have minimal anticholinergic effects. Doxepin, dothiepin, maprotiline, nomifensine, and trazodone are least cardiotoxic.

Clomipramine is claimed to be specifically effective in obsessive–compulsive neurosis when depressed mood is present.

Nomifensine has dopaminergic activity and is recommended if depression coexists with Parkinsonism.

MONOAMINE OXIDASE INHIBITORS (MAOIs) (Table 2)

Indications (Tyrer, 1976)

1. Depressive neurosis, including mixed depressive/anxiety neurosis.

2. Phobic anxiety states.
3. Depressive illness which has failed to respond to tricyclics.

Pharmacology

MAOIs increase concentration of monoamines, including neurotransmitters in the brain and other amines elsewhere in the body, by inhibiting the enzyme concerned in their breakdown.

Administration

MAOIs may need to be given for up to three weeks before their full effect is apparent. They can be started in a small dose which is increased as tolerance to side-effects develops. They are given in two or three doses daily, or in a single morning dose if this does not produce side-effects.

Side-effects

1. *Neurological and psychiatric:* insomnia, drowsiness, excitement or mania, peripheral neuropathy.

2. *Cardiovascular:* postural hypotension, oedema.

3. *Gastrointestinal:* dry mouth, nausea, constipation.

4. *Endocrine and metabolic:* weight gain.

5. *Ocular:* blurred vision.

6. *Genitourinary:* difficulty in micturition, sexual dysfunction.

7. *Other:* hepatocellular jaundice, sweating, rash.

Contraindications

Liver disease, cardiac failure.

Tolerance and Dependence

Psychological dependence may occur.

Metabolism

MAOIs are probably metabolized to inactive compounds by acetylation in the liver. This occurs more rapidly in some people than others, ('slow and fast acetylators'), the difference being genetically determined, but it is not known whether acetylator status predicts clinical response.

Drug and Food Interactions

Hypertensive crisis, occasionally fatal, may result if MAOIs are combined with sympathomimetic drugs or tyramine-containing foods.

The drugs concerned include amphetamines, L-dopa, fenfluramine, local anaesthetics, ephedrine and related drugs (often found in proprietary cough and cold cures).

Strong cheese and red wine, especially Chianti, are the most important of a long list of foods which may cause reactions. Preserved protein foods like smoked fish and hung game, and protein extracts like 'Marmite', are others.

Potentiation of hypoglycaemics, opiates, barbiturates, anticholinergics, hypotensives, tricyclic antidepressants, phenytoin, and alcohol may occur.

Enhanced therapeutic effects may be obtained by combining MAOIs with a tricyclic antidepressant or with L-tryptophan. The combination with tricyclics carries a risk of hypertensive crisis, and should be started in hospital using small doses.

Choice of Drug

Phenelzine is most widely used. Isocarboxazid is more sedative, and tranylcypromine more stimulant.

BENZODIAZEPINES (Table 3)

Benzodiazepines are very widely prescribed as anxiolytics and hypnotics. About 6% of the population take them.

Indications

1. Anxiety.
2. Insomnia.
3. Alcohol withdrawal states.
4. Status epilepticus.
5. Muscle spasticity.

Table 3 Benzodiazepines

Short-acting
Lorazepam (Ativan)
Lormetazepam (Noctamid)
Oxazepam (Serenid)
Temazepam (Normison, Euhypnos)
Triazolam (Halcion)

Long-acting
Chlordiazepoxide (Librium)
Clobazam (Frisium)
Clonazepam (Rivotril)
Clorazepate (Tranxene)
Diazepam (Valium)
Flurazepam (Dalmane)
Ketazolam (Anxon)
Medazepam (Nobrium)
Nitrazepam (Mogadon)

Pharmacology

Benzodiazepines probably act through modification of the GABA and glycine neurotransmitter systems in the limbic system and spinal cord.

Administration

Benzodiazepines used for anxiety or insomnia are more effective if taken only as required, rather than on a fixed dose regimen, and for periods of not more than a few weeks at a time.

Side-effects

Benzodiazepines have few unwanted effects, even in overdose, in the young healthy person, but the elderly may experience marked side-effects which include:

1. *Neurological and psychiatric:* confusion, depression, drowsiness (but in a few subjects 'paradoxical' effects of excitement, aggression or insomnia), impaired psychomotor performance, ataxia, dysarthria, headache.

2. *Cardiovascular:* hypotension.

3. *Gastrointestinal:* nausea, constipation.

4. *Endocrine and metabolic:* weight gain, mild hypothyroidism.

5. *Ocular:* blurred vision, glaucoma.

6. *Genitourinary:* retention or incontinence of urine.

7. *Allergic:* rash.

8. *Others:* mild teratogenic effects such as cleft palate have been reported if benzodiazepines are used in early pregnancy.

Tolerance and Dependence

Tolerance develops with regular use. Psychological dependence is common. Physical dependence is rare, but may develop if large doses are taken, in which case suddenly stopping the drug causes a withdrawal syndrome of insomnia, tremor, fits, vomiting, sweating, and cramps.

Drug Interactions

Benzodiazepines potentiate the effects of alcohol and other cerebral depressants.

Choice of Drug

Many benzodiazepines are available. The differences between them concern potency and duration of action. Several of them are metabolized to the same compound, oxazepam. Any of them can be used in low dose for treating anxiety, or in high dose for treating insomnia. The short-acting ones, for which the plasma half-life of the drug and its active metabolites is less than 10 hours, are suitable for insomnia which is not accompanied by anxiety, or for phobic anxiety which lasts a short time in certain situations. The longer-acting ones can be given in a single daily dose at night, providing both an immediate hypnotic effect and an anxiolytic effect next day.

LITHIUM (Ghose, 1977)

Lithium is the lightest of the alkali metals.

Indications

1. Prophylaxis of affective disorder in patients whose attacks are

frequent or severe enough to justify continuous treatment; at least three attacks in two years. It is effective in the majority of patients, but probably more effective in bipolar than unipolar disease.
2. Treatment of mania.
3. Suggested uses awaiting evaluation include treatment of established depression, behaviour disturbance from various causes, alcoholism, tardive dyskinesia, migraine, blood disorders, and thyroid disease.

Pharmacology

The mode of action of lithium in preventing affective disorders is unknown, but it has the following physiological properties.

1. Cerebral sodium concentration and bone mineral content are reduced.
2. Monoamine synthesis is increased, as is the uptake of 5-HT by platelets.
3. Cyclic AMP is inhibited.
4. Endocrine effects are reduction of thyroid hormone synthesis because of enzyme inhibition, and a consequent increase of TSH secretion; increase of aldosterone secretion; increase of antidiuretic hormone secretion.
5. The distal tubules of the kidneys become insensitive to antidiuretic hormone, causing nephrogenic diabetes insipidus.

Administration

Lithium is usually given as the carbonate, but any one of its soluble salts (citrate, sulphate, monoglutamate, or acetate) may be used instead. Only oral preparations are available.

Plain lithium carbonate is given three times daily to produce a steady serum level. Slow release tablets for once daily administration are available, but even these give a peak serum level soon after administration.

Therapeutic effect is related to serum lithium level. This should be 0.8–1.2 mmol/litre for prophylaxis of affective disorder, and 1.2–2.0 mmol/litre for treatment of mania. There is some individual variation in the level required for therapeutic effect, and in dosage needed to produce a particular serum level. Serum level must be measured at a fixed interval, conventionally 8 hours, after the last dose. Toxic effects are usual when the level exceeds 2.0 mmol/litre but may develop at lower levels.

Serum lithium level should be measured weekly for the first 4 weeks of treatment, then monthly for a year, and then every 3 months. It should also be measured in the event of intercurrent illness, or if symptoms suggesting lithium toxicity develop.

Thyroid, renal, and cardiac function should be assessed before starting treatment, and then annually.

The therapeutic effect in mania may be delayed for a week or more, and the prophylactic effect in affective disorder may be delayed for some months.

If a patient has remained free of attacks of affective disorder for some years, it is reasonable to try withdrawing lithium, as the disease may have undergone a natural remission and continuing lithium indefinitely may be unnecessary and may produce irreversible side-effects.

Side-effects

1. *Relatively harmless:* nausea, mild diarrhoea, fine tremor (which can be treated by a beta blocker), weight gain, oedema, and exacerbation of psoriasis.

2. *Serious:*

(a) Acute symptoms suggesting lithium intoxication are vomiting, diarrhoea, coarse tremor, drowsiness, vertigo, dysarthria, and cardiac arrhythmias. If any of these develop, lithium should be stopped, and blood taken for estimation of the serum level.

(b) Long-term effects of gradual onset are hypothyroidism (affecting 3% of cases per year, usually reversible when lithium is stopped, and treatable with thyroxine if lithium is continued); nephrogenic diabetes insipidus (manifest by thirst and polyuria); depletion of calcium in bone; and possibly memory impairment. Thyrotoxicosis rather than hypothyroidism has occasionally been reported.

Contraindications

Lithium should be avoided, or used in low dose with close supervision, in patients who have cardiac or renal impairment, thyroid disease, diabetes insipidus, Addison's disease, are obese, or are taking diuretics. Neurological impairment after combined treatment with lithium and haloperidol in high doses has been reported. Lithium is best avoided during pregnancy since it may cause minor congenital abnormalities, hypothyroidism, and impaired bone development; it should also be avoided during breast-feeding since it enters breast milk.

Further Reading

Recommended books on psychopharmacology are those by Crammer *et al.* (1978) and by Silverstone and Turner (1978). The relevant sections in the general pharmacology book by Goodman and Gilman (1975) are also useful.

References

Crammer, J., Barraclough, B., and Heine, B. (1978). *The Use of Drugs in Psychiatry*. Gaskell, London.
Ghose, K. (1977). Lithium salts: therapeutic and unwanted effects. *Br. J. Hosp. Med.* **18**, 578–583.
Goodman, L. S. and Gilman, A. (Eds.) (1975). *The Pharmacological Basis of Therapeutics*. Macmillan, New York.
Mackay, A. V. P., and Sheppard, G. P. (1979). Pharmacotherapeutic trials in tardive dyskinesia. *Br. J. Psychiatry*, **135**, 489–499.
Silverstone, T., and Turner, P. (1978). *Drug Treatment in Psychiatry*. Routledge and Kegan Paul, London.
Tyrer, P. (1976). Towards rational therapy with monoamine oxidase inhibitors. *Br. J. Psychiatry*, **128**, 354–360.

CHAPTER 21

Other Physical Treatment Methods

ECT (ELECTROCONVULSIVE THERAPY)

ECT involves production of a fit by passing an electric current through the brain.

Artificially induced fits have been used in treating mental illness since the eighteenth century. Chemicals, including intravenous leptazol (Metrazol) and inhalation of flurothyl (Indoklon), are an alternative means of producing fits, but electricity is more controllable. Modern ECT was introduced by Cerletti in 1938. During the 1950s the procedure was refined by the addition of a muscle relaxant to reduce the intensity of the fit, and of short-acting anaesthesia to reduce the patient's distress.

Indications

1. Depressive illness: ECT is usually given in preference to drugs

(a) to produce a rapid antidepressant response in patients who are suicidal, or refusing to eat or drink;
(b) when tricyclic drugs are contraindicated for medical reasons e.g. cardiac arrhythmias;
(c) when drugs have failed.

Features predicting a good response (Carney *et al.*, 1965) are those characteristic of depressive psychosis: severe depression, retardation, guilt, delusions, early wakening, symptoms worse in the morning, short duration of illness, and good premorbid personality. Features predicting a poor response are those characteristic of depressive neurosis: anxiety, hypochondriasis, hysterical symptoms, and neurotic premorbid personality. Depressive neurosis may be made worse by ECT.

2. Schizophrenia which has failed to respond to drugs.
3. Catatonic schizophrenia.
4. Mania which has failed to respond to drugs.

Efficacy and Mode of Action

Of patients with depressive illness, 70-80% respond to ECT. The response rates in schizophrenia and mania are not known.

The mode of action is unknown, although possibilities include:

1. biochemical changes: increased efficiency of monoamine pathways (Grahame-Smith *et al.*, 1978), increased prolactin production.
2. a powerful placebo effect resulting from the complexity of the treatment, the mystique surrounding it, and the extra medical and nursing attention.
3. the memory loss is therapeutic.

It is not clear whether a fit is necessary for a therapeutic effect, or even whether the electric shock is necessary. Several recent trials have compared ECT with 'pseudo-ECT' in which an anaesthetic and muscle relaxant are given, but no electric shock; the largest (Johnstone *et al.*, 1980) found that depressed patients improved with either treatment, but those given 'real' ECT improved more quickly. Taylor and Fleminger (1980) obtained similar results in patients with paranoid schizophrenia.

Number and Spacing of Treatments

The number of treatments required to produce a response varies considerably, but in most cases there is improvement after two or three treatments and about six are needed in all. If there is no improvement after six treatments, there is probably no point in continuing the course. ECT is given two or three times a week in depressive illness, and more frequent administration has no advantage. Daily treatment may be more effective for mania and schizophrenia.

Bilateral and Unilateral ECT (d'Elia and Raotma, 1975)

The electrodes may be applied to both sides of the head (bilateral ECT), or to the side of the non-dominant hemisphere only (unilateral ECT). Bilateral ECT produces more memory loss and confusion in the short term, but is more effective in that fewer treatments per course are needed when bilateral ECT is used.

Side-effects

1. *Memory impairment:* transient memory impairment, both retrograde and anterograde, is frequent. A few patients complain of persistent

memory damage, but cognitive testing several months after ECT shows only mild impairment which is no worse than that found in depressives treated by other means (Weeks *et al.*, 1980).

2. *Confusion:* mild transient confusion after treatment is frequent. If a severe confusional state occurs, the patient probably has brain damage, and treatment should be stopped.

3. *Anaesthetic complications.*

4. *Fractures:* not a hazard when the fit is adequately modified by a muscle relaxant.

5. *Mania* may be precipitated when ECT is given to patients with bipolar affective disorder in the depressed phase.

Mortality is 1 per 30,000 treatments, virtually always from anaesthetic complications.

Contraindications

1. Anaesthetic contraindications, e.g. cardiac or respiratory disease.
2. Organic brain disease, including dementia, which may become worse after ECT or be temporarily complicated by an acute confusional state.

The presence of contraindications may need to be balanced against the risk to life entailed by severe depression when deciding whether ECT is justified.

Further Reading

Detailed accounts are given by Clare (1980a) and Freeman (1979).

PSYCHOSURGERY
(LEUCOTOMY, FUNCTIONAL NEUROSURGERY)

Definition

Brain surgery carried out in order to relieve suffering by changing mood or behaviour.

History

Moniz introduced psychosurgery in 1936. The 'standard leucotomy', involving extensive division of frontolimbic connections, was carried out on thousands of patients during the next 20 years. However, it became clear that most did not benefit, and deaths and side-effects were common. When effective drug treatments became available in the 1950s the operation was virtually abandoned, and in some countries banned by legislation, but interest in psychosurgery revived when more sophisticated neurosurgical techniques were developed. About 100–200 operations are carried out annually in England and Wales at present.

Techniques

Modern operations usually use stereotactic methods for location of small target areas. Lesions may be made by cutting, freezing, thermocoagulation, radioisotopes, or suction. Sites include the frontal lobe, temporal lobe, cingulum, amygdala, thalamus, and hypothalamus. There is incomplete agreement about the indications for selecting any particular site.

Indications

Psychosurgery is reserved for severe, long-standing cases of mental illness or behaviour disorder which have failed to respond to any other treatment. Depression, anxiety and obsessive–compulsive symptoms respond best. Psychosurgery is also sometimes used for schizophrenia, anorexia nervosa, and control of repeated violence or sexual offences.

Efficacy

A controlled trial has not been done because of practical and ethical objections. The success rate in uncontrolled trials is 70–80% in depression, anxiety, and obsessive–compulsive neurosis, is much lower in schizophrenia, and has not been evaluated in other conditions.

Contraindications

1. Sociopathic personality traits, and drug or alcohol abuse, which may get worse after the operation because of the disinhibition it may cause.

2. Dementia, which may be exacerbated.
3. Physical contraindications, e.g. hypertension, haemorrhagic tendencies.
4. Absence of informed consent.

Side-effects

Mortality and morbidity were high after the early leucotomies. Modern operations have a negligible mortality, but cause side-effects in up to 10% of patients: disinhibition, lethargy, epilepsy, intellectual defects, neurological symptoms, incontinence, weight gain, and endocrine changes.

Further Reading

Detailed accounts are given in the book by Clare (1980b), and in the review article by Schurr (1973).

References

Carney, M. W. P., Roth, M., and Garside, R. F. (1965). The diagnosis of depressive syndromes and the prediction of ECT response. *Br. J. Psychiatry*, **111**, 659–674.

Clare, A. (1980a). Electroconvulsive therapy. In *Psychiatry in Dissent*. Tavistock, London.

Clare, A. (1980b). Psychosurgery. In *Psychiatry in Dissent*. Tavistock, London.

d'Elia, G., and Raotma, H. (1975). Is unilateral ECT less effective than bilateral ECT? *Br. J. Psychiatry*, **126**, 83–89.

Freeman, C. P. L. (1979). Electroconvulsive therapy: its current clinical use. *Br. J. Hosp. Med.*, **21**, 281–292.

Grahame-Smith, D. G., Green, A. R., and Costain, D. W. (1978). Mechanism of the antidepressant action of ECT. *Lancet*. **i**, 254.

Johnstone, E., Deakin, J. F. W., Lawler, P., Frith, C. D., Stevens, M., McPherson, K., and Crow, T. J. (1980). The Northwick Park electroconvulsive therapy trial. *Lancet*, **ii**, 1317–1320.

Schurr, P. (1973). Psychosurgery. *Br. J. Hosp. Med.* **10**, 53–60.

Taylor, P., and Fleminger, J. J. (1980). ECT for schizophrenia. *Lancet* **i**, 1380–1383.

Weeks, D., Freeman, C. P. L., and Kendell, R. E. (1980). ECT:III. Enduring cognitive deficits? *Br. J. Psychiatry*, **137**, 26–37.

CHAPTER 22

Psychological Treatment Methods

PRINCIPLES OF PSYCHOTHERAPY

Psychotherapy utilizes the interaction between patient and therapist to achieve changes in the patient's emotions and behaviour.

Psychotherapy may be divided into supportive and psychodynamic types. In supportive psychotherapy the therapist's role is that of sympathetic listener and adviser, and the patient's problems are discussed at a relatively simple, practical level. It may be combined with other forms of treatment. Counselling, e.g. marriage guidance, is a form of supportive psychotherapy which was developed to help psychiatrically normal people with problems caused by difficult life situations. Psychodynamic (analytic, exploratory, intensive) psychotherapy is a more ambitious treatment in which the aim is to achieve lasting personality changes.

Psychotherapy may be carried out with individuals, couples, families, or groups, and in the style of one of many schools.

Selection of Patient and Therapist

The most suitable patients are those suffering from neurotic symptoms or mild personality disorders who are well motivated to change, firmly committed to treatment, able to understand psychological concepts, prepared to take responsibility for decisions, and are reasonably young, intelligent, and verbally fluent. Patients who have psychotic illnesses, are taking large quantities of drugs or alcohol, or have severe personality disorders are usually considered unsuitable.

Desirable qualities in a therapist are the ability to be sympathetic but detached, non-judgmental, and honest. Therapy is more likely to be successful if patient and therapist like one another.

Mechanisms of Change

Increased self-esteem and improvement of symptoms may result solely from the opportunity to have a reliable and sympathetic relationship with the therapist, as emphasized by Rogers (1951) in his system of 'client-centred' therapy. More profound personality changes may be achieved if the patient can acquire insight into maladaptive behaviour patterns, and the reasons for these, through the therapist's interpretations. Intellectual insight usually occurs first, but needs to be followed by emotional change, and applied to real life situations, if it is to be valuable.

Planning and Organization of Therapy

Treatment sessions usually take place weekly and last an hour, and the duration of treatment is months or years. Some therapists draw up a 'contract' at the beginning to specify the patient's problems, goals of treatment, and the proposed number and timing of sessions.

Evaluation of Results

Numerous studies show that most patients improve after psychotherapy, but it is not clear whether improvement is the result of the treatment itself, of the spontaneous remission often seen in neurotic disorders, or a non-specific effect of the close individual attention which patients receive. Difficulties in the evaluation of results include:

1. Many patients given psychotherapy do not fit into conventional diagnostic categories.
2. The content of treatment sessions cannot be standardized since it varies with the individual characteristics of patient and therapist.
3. There is no adequate form of 'placebo' psychotherapy which could be given to a control group.
4. The criteria by which outcome should be measured are not agreed.

Unwanted Effects of Psychotherapy

1. Patients may become excessively dependent on therapy or the therapist.
2. Intensive psychotherapy may be distressing to the patient and result in exacerbation of symptoms, and deterioration in relationships.
3. Some psychotherapists are not trained to recognise disorders for which physical treatments would be more appropriate, e.g. psychotic states, or physical illness presenting with mental symptoms.
4. Ineffective psychotherapy wastes time and money, and damages patients' morale.

GROUP THERAPY (Ryle, 1976)

Group therapy is preferable to individual therapy for some patients, and is economical of therapist time.

Selection of Patients

Criteria for selection are similar to those for psychotherapy in general.

Group therapy may benefit patients whose main problems concern relationships with others, and patients with a shared problem such as alcoholism, drug addiction, or sociopathy. Very shy patients who find it difficult to participate in group discussion may not benefit, whereas very talkative patients may monopolize a group and arouse hostility, but a skilled therapist may encourage both types of patient to play a more balanced role. Careful selection is important since 'dropping-out' damages morale both for patients who leave and those who stay.

Role of the Therapist

The therapist should discourage factors likely to impede the group's success, e.g. dropping-out, lateness, absences, socialization outside the group, and sub-grouping.

Some therapists act as detached leaders, others participate more actively. Large groups may have two cotherapists, preferably of equal status. Occasional meetings without a leader may be successful if a group is well established.

Mechanisms of Change

Yalom (1975) has listed the following curative factors in group therapy: catharsis, self-disclosure, learning from interpersonal actions, universality, acceptance, altruism, guidance, self-understanding, vicarious learning, and instillation of hope.

Organization of Therapy

As the introduction of newcomers may retard progress and arouse hostility, 'closed' groups with a fixed life span and the same members throughout are ideal, though not always practicable. The ideal size is 5–10 patients. Outpatient groups usually meet weekly for 1–2 hours for 1–2 years. Inpatient units run on 'therapeutic community' lines (Clark, 1965) use daily group therapy as the sole method of treatment.

Individual therapy may be combined with group therapy if a patient is under special stress.

FAMILY THERAPY (Skynner, 1976)

The rationale for family therapy is the belief that psychiatric symptoms are sometimes exacerbated or even caused by dysfunction within the patient's family. Types of dysfunction which may be treated by family therapy include 'scapegoating', in which one member is blamed for all the family problems; excessive authority or dependency of certain members; ambiguous styles of communication; gratification of one member through the illness of another; and situations in which a shared stress, e.g. bereavement, is affecting more than one member.

The therapist, after observing the family together, helps its members to examine and change such abnormal patterns of interaction.

Prerequisites for a successful outcome are thought to be the existence of a defined family group, motivation towards improvement in all its members, and some degree of goodwill and honesty between them.

SCHOOLS OF PSYCHOTHERAPY

Sigmund Freud (1856–1939)

Freud's system of 'psychoanalysis' forms the basis of most modern forms of psychodynamic psychotherapy. During psychoanalysis (in which treatment sessions lasting 50 minutes each take place 3–5 times a week for several years) the patient talks about past and present events, emotions, dreams, and fantasies, and uses 'free association' from these to recall repressed or forgotten material to conscious awareness. The therapist's interpretations relate to Freud's concepts which include:

1. transference, a phenomenon in which the patient experiences inappropriate emotions towards the therapist, derived from emotions felt towards other people in the past. (Countertransference is the equivalent experience of inappropriate emotions by the therapist towards the patient.)
2. resistance, in which the patient avoids exploration of a topic which is the subject of unconscious conflicts.
3. ego defence mechanisms, which are unconscious processes to reduce anxiety, and include denial, repression, rationalization, projection, reaction formation, displacement, sublimation, intellectualization, conversion, fixation, regression, and introjection (see Glossary).
4. dreams, in which the real or 'latent' content is converted into the 'manifest' content by the mental 'censor' using the mechanisms of condensation, displacement, and symbolism.

5. 'parapraxes', the mistakes and forgetfulness of everyday life which have unconscious significance.
6. stages of psychosexual development: oral, anal, genital, and oedipal; in each of which the libido, or sexual energy, is attached in a particular direction ('cathexis').
7. psychic structure, which may be conceptualized as the id (inherited, instinctive, largely unconscious, motivated by the 'pleasure principle'), the ego (largely conscious, acting according to the 'reality principle', and using the ego defence mechanisms), and the superego (derived from introjection of authority figures, and equivalent to conscience). An alternative way of conceptualizing psychic structure is to divide it into the conscious, preconscious, and unconscious.
8. the repetition compulsion, and the death wish (thanatos).

Freud's theories are summarized by Stafford-Clark (1967).

Carl Jung (1875-1961)

Jung's system of psychotherapy is called analytical psychology. It emphasizes the exploration of dreams and the unconscious, and aims at 'individuation' of the patient; this involves achieving harmony between the conscious and unconscious, and full experience of the self. Jungian concepts include:

1. libido, or general psychic energy, flowing between pairs of opposites such as progression–regression, conscious–unconscious, extraversion–introversion. If it is blocked in one direction pathology results, e.g. excess energy in the unconscious manifest as psychiatric illness.
2. the unconscious mind, as revealed in dreams, with both personal and collective aspects, the latter including instincts, archetypes, and universal symbols.
3. personality depends on the degree of extraversion or introversion, and on which of the 'four functions'—thinking, feeling, sensation and intuition—is most highly developed. There is an outward personality, or 'persona', and an unconscious 'shadow' which has opposite characteristics.

Jung's theories are summarized by Storr (1973).

Alfred Adler (1870-1937)

Adler's system of psychotherapy is called 'individual psychology' and uses an easily understood, commonsense approach.

Adler considered that the basic force in life is the wish to rise from inferiority to superiority in the fields of work and personal relationships, so gaining self-esteem, approval, and material success. People who feel inferior because of physical defects or psychological handicaps may either fail to compensate, compensate successfully, or overcompensate and have an exaggerated opinion of their own abilities. He used the term 'life-style' to describe a person's interaction with the environment. He viewed neurosis as a means of gaining attention and escaping responsibility by adopting the role of a sick person.

Melanie Klein (1882–1960)

Klein worked with children under 2 years old, and believed that failure of psychological development at this time was the origin of neurosis in later life. She described developmental stages, the 'paranoid position' and the 'depressive position', related to the child's perception of its mother's breast first as a 'good' object which is introjected, and then as a 'bad' object on to which aggressive feelings are projected. Klein's theories are summarized by Segal (1979).

Other 'neo-Freudians' include Fromm, Reich, Erikson, Sullivan, Horney, Anna Freud, Winnicot, and Fairburn (Brown, 1961). There are many more recent schools of psychotherapy, too numerous to summarize here; they tend to differ from traditional methods in that treatment is less prolonged, the therapist plays a more active role, and actions are used as well as words (Aveline, 1979).

Further Reading

Short general books on psychotherapy are those by Bloch (1979) and Brown and Pedder (1979).

BEHAVIOUR THERAPY

Modern behaviour therapy was started in the 1950s. Names associated with its development include Eysenck, Lazarus, Wolpe, Bandura, Marks, and Rachman.

Behaviour therapy is based on learning theory, and was originally applied to those neurotic symptoms which could be regarded as 'maladaptive learned responses', but has since been applied to a wider range of disorders.

Improved behaviour may entail either the loss of symptoms, or the acquisition of desirable new behaviour.

The patient's problems are defined, and objectives of therapy agreed at the beginning. Progress during treatment is measured as accurately as possible using such criteria as the frequency of occurrence of a particular behaviour pattern, questionnaires to monitor mood changes, or psycho-physiological variables.

Present symptoms are emphasized, rather than past events or unconscious conflicts. This lack of attention to underlying causes has led to criticism that behaviour therapy cannot effect a real cure, as relief of one symptom will result in its replacement by another. In practice this 'symptom substitution' is uncommon.

Behaviour therapy is at least equal in efficacy to other forms of psychotherapy, often less time-consuming than other methods, and the patient need not be intelligent or verbally fluent to benefit. It was developed by psychologists but can be carried out by psychiatrists or nurses with appropriate training. Behaviour therapy and drug treatment can be usefully combined.

The main conditions in which behaviour therapy may be useful, and the techniques used to treat them, are listed below.

1. *Phobic anxiety states:*
   (a) Systematic desensitization (Lipsedge, 1973): relaxation training is combined with gradual exposure to the feared stimulus, over several sessions in which the stimulus is presented in a progressively anxiety-provoking form.
   (b) Flooding (implosion): the patient is immediately exposed to the feared stimulus in its most intense form.
   (c) Modelling: the patient imitates the therapist in dealing with the feared stimulus. Modelling can be combined with other methods.

Behaviour therapy is the treatment of choice for monophobias, which are easier to treat than generalized phobic states.

2. *Anxiety states with prominent somatic symptoms:*
   (a) Muscular relaxation training.
   (b) Biofeedback techniques to modify physiological variables, e.g. heart rate, blood pressure, and muscle tension.

3. *Obsessive–compulsive disorders* (Beech, 1978):
   (a) Response prevention, including thought stopping.
   (b) Massed practice, or satiation.

Behaviour therapy is the treatment of choice.

4. *Undesirable behaviour*, e.g. deviant sexuality, excess drinking, eating, smoking, or gambling, and certain repeated criminal behaviour:

(a) Aversion therapy: performance of the undesirable behaviour is coupled with an unpleasant stimulus such as an electric shock. This treatment appears to be effective, but is now seldom used because of ethical criticisms. It should never be used without the patient's informed consent.

(b) Covert sensitization: the patient is made aware of the likely unpleasant consequences of his behaviour by suggestion only.

(c) Encouragement of more desirable alternative forms of behaviour.

5. *Teaching basic skills*, and encouraging socially acceptable behaviour, in mentally handicapped (Chapter 19) or chronically institutionalized patients:

(a) Shaping, or chaining: learning each stage in a complex process like dressing is rewarded as it occurs.

(b) Token economy regimens: patients receive rewards for desirable behaviour, but have privileges withdrawn for undesirable behaviour.

6. *Treatment of sexual dysfunction* (Chapter 12).

7. *Social skills training* (Argyle, 1972).

Further Reading

Review articles on behaviour therapy by Chesser (1976) and Marks (1976a,b).

References

Argyle, M. (1972). *Psychology of Interpersonal Behaviour*. Penguin, Harmondsworth.

Aveline, M. (1979). Action techniques in psychotherapy. *Br. J. Hosp. Med.*, **22**, 78–84.

Beech, H. R. (1978). Advances in the treatment of obsessional neurosis. *Br. J. Hosp. Med.*, **19**, 54–60.

Bloch, S. (Ed.) (1979). *An Introduction to the Psychotherapies*. Oxford University Press, Oxford.

Brown, D., and Pedder, J. (1979). *An Introduction to Psychotherapy*. Tavistock Publications, London.

Brown, J. A. C. (1961). *Freud and the Post-Freudians*. Penguin, Harmondsworth.

Chesser, E. S. (1976). Behaviour therapy: recent trends and current practice. *Br. J. Psychiatry*, **129**, 289–307.

Clark, D. H. (1965). The therapeutic community—concept, practice and future. *Br. J. Psychiatry*, **111**, 947–954.

Lipsedge, M. S. (1973). Systematic desensitisation in phobic disorders. *Br. J. Hosp. Med.*, **9**, 657–664.

Marks, I. M. (1976a). The current status of behavioural psychotherapy: theory and practice. *Am. J. Psychiatry*, **133**, 253–261.

Marks, I. M. (1976b). Behavioural psychotherapy. *Br. J. Hosp. Med.*, **15**, 250–256.

Rogers, C. R. (1951). *Client-Centred Therapy*. Houghton Mifflin, Boston.

Ryle, A. (1976). Group psychotherapy. *Br. J. Hosp. Med.*, **15**, 239–248.

Segal, H. (1979). *Klein*. Fontana, London.

Skynner, A. C. R. (1976). Family and marital psychotherapy. *Br. J. Hosp. Med.*, **15**, 224–234.

Stafford-Clark, D. (1967). *What Freud Really Said*. Penguin, Harmondsworth.

Storr, A. (1973). *Jung*. Fontana, London.

Yalom, I. D. (1975). *The Theory and Practice of Group Psychotherapy*. Basic Books, New York.

CHAPTER 23

Social Aspects of Psychiatry

EPIDEMIOLOGY

Epidemiology is the study of morbidity and mortality rates, their trends over time, and their variation with other factors, in defined populations.

Epidemiological research enables:

1. evaluation of treatment, and treatment facilities.
2. prediction of the nature and extent of future treatment services likely to be required.
3. detection of new cases in the community.
4. identification of factors associated with particular conditions, which may be important in their aetiology.
5. fuller description of clinical syndromes, and refinements of classification for 'functional' conditions which are diagnosed on the basis of their symptoms and natural history.

Before a condition can be studied it must be defined in reproducible terms. For conditions in which there is no clear distinction between 'cases' and 'normals', e.g. neuroses, personality disorders, and alcoholism, it is necessary to choose a 'boundary of severity' to define the degree of abnormality which is clinically significant.

Cross-sectional surveys examine the prevalence of illness at a point in time. Longitudinal surveys, prospective or retrospective, follow trends over time. Longitudinal surveys provide more information, including incidence rates, and data on the natural history of disease; but prospective studies may take years to complete, and retrospective ones are often impeded by inadequate or inaccurate data.

The sources of information for surveys include:

1. planned inquiries, in which every member of a defined population, or a random sample of it, is investigated by interview or questionnaire. A widely used screening instrument for this purpose is the General

Health Questionnaire (GHQ) (Goldberg, 1972) designed to detect neurotic symptoms.
2. GP consultation records.
3. case registers, specially designed to record all contacts with psychiatric services.
4. hospital statistics.

Different sources yield different morbidity rates. Community surveys detect the highest rates, and hospital statistics the lowest. Variations in rates derived from hospital statistics may reflect differences in treatment policy rather than true changes in the frequency of disease.

Results may be expressed as prevalence rates, including point prevalence for the day of inquiry, and period prevalence over a time span such as one year; incidence rates; and lifetime expectancy. One or other method may be more appropriate for a given condition depending on whether it is acute, chronic or episodic, rare or common.

Different studies have produced varying estimates of frequency for the same conditions, because of differences in the definition of cases, the data sources, and the mode of expressing the results. A survey in London (Shepherd *et al.*, 1966) showed that 14% of the population consulted their GP for psychiatric symptoms during one year.

Social Correlates of Illness

Surveys can provide information about social variables associated with illness by comparing illness rates in populations with different social characteristics (ecological surveys), or by comparing the social characteristics of 'cases' with those of the rest of the population.

The social factors which correlate with psychiatric illness are not necessarily causal. They may operate indirectly by influencing the likelihood of referral or hospitalization, or may be the result rather than the cause of the illness.

1. *Social class:* the rates for most conditions, with the exception of affective disorders, suicide, and alcoholism, are higher in social classes IV and V, despite the greater likelihood of specialist referral for patients in classes I and II. Possible explanations are:

(a) mental illness prevents advancement and causes downward social drift.

(b) the social stresses to which classes IV and V are prone cause illness.

(c) there is greater genetic predisposition to illness in classes IV and V.

2. *Marital status:* morbidity rates in men are highest for the divorced and lowest for the married, with the widowed and single in between. Possible explanations are:

(a) the stress of divorce or bereavement precipitates illness.

(b) people who have, or are predisposed to develop, psychiatric illness, either do not marry at all, or have unsuccessful marriages leading to divorce.

(c) a successful marriage protects against illness.

Young married women, however, have higher rates of neurotic illness than single ones.

3. *Residential area:* morbidity rates are higher in urban than rural districts, being especially high in poor areas of big cities. Possible explanations are:

(a) the mentally ill move into poor city areas because of their cheapness and anonymity.

(b) the stress of life in such areas causes mental illness. Social isolation and disorganization are believed to be most important.

4. *Nationality:* rates for the psychoses are similar in different countries, but rates for alcoholism, suicide, homicide and 'culture-bound' syndromes vary.

5. *Life events:* major environmental stresses have often been observed to precipitate psychiatric illness, e.g. a very high incidence of acute neurotic breakdown is found among fighting troops in wartime. The impact of life events has recently been studied extensively (Editorial, 1978). Patients with schizophrenia, depression, and acute neurosis are more likely than those with physical illnesses or healthy controls to have experienced life events before becoming ill. Unpleasant events account for the excess, and events causing loss are especially implicated in precipitating depression. Most of the studies have been retrospective. Problems in interpreting the results of life event research include:

(a) an event apparently preceding an illness might in fact result from the patient's altered behaviour during the unrecognized prodromal phase.

(b) the importance of life events may be exaggerated by patients or relatives in an attempt to find the explanation for becoming ill ('effort after meaning').

(c) definable, datable events are emphasized, but chronic stresses could be equally important.

(d) it is difficult to generalize about which incidents should be accorded the status of 'life events', or how much weight to attach to each type of event, since the same one, e.g. a change of job, might have far more significance for some people than others.

(e) depressive illness has to be distinguished from simple unhappiness after an unpleasant life event.

Most people experience unpleasant life events without becoming ill, but life events may precipitate illness in predisposed people; mathematical formulae for 'relative risk' and 'brought forward time' have been proposed to quantify this effect.

6. *Social influence:* 'epidemics' of hysterical symptoms or of suicide by particular methods can occur in communities. Mental illness in one individual may precipitate illness in other family members.

PREVENTION

Primary prevention is prevention of disease from ever developing. It includes:

1. medical and public health measures to avert conditions with an organic aetiology:
   (a) genetic counselling, and amniocentesis followed by abortion if necessary;
   (b) improved health of pregnant mothers, e.g. avoidance of alcohol, drugs and smoking;
   (c) improved obstetric care, e.g. to avoid birth injury;
   (d) improved infant welfare services, e.g. immunizations;
   (e) emergency treatment of infantile convulsions to prevent temporal lobe epilepsy;
   (f) control and early treatment of infections, e.g. syphilis, meningitis, at any age;
   (g) avoidance of nutritional deficiencies;
   (h) reduction of alcohol consumption;
   (i) reduction of environmental pollution, e.g. atmospheric lead;

(j) prevention of accidents, and hence of head injury, e.g. by seat belts and crash helmets;
2. psychological approaches:
   (a) counselling for the bereaved, divorced, and other groups known to have a high risk of illness;
   (b) crisis intervention;
   (c) social work with disturbed families, with particular emphasis on avoiding adverse effects on their children.

The preventive value of such measures is not established.

Secondary prevention is reduction of the severity of established disease by means of early detection and treatment.

Tertiary prevention is the reduction of the indirect consequences of established disease, e.g. prevention of institutionalization by rehabilitation, and relief of the burden on patients' families by community services.

Further Reading

Epidemiology as applied to psychiatry is discussed in the books by Cooper and Morgan (1973) and Hare and Wing (1970).

TRANSCULTURAL PSYCHIATRY (Cox, 1977)

Transcultural psychiatry includes the comparative study of different cultures with respect to the type and prevalence of mental illness within them, and study of the psychiatric aspects of immigration.

Investigation of the subject is complicated by language barriers, the lack of internationally agreed criteria for diagnosing psychiatric illness, and the influence cultural background may have on symptomatology and its interpretation.

Culture-specific Syndromes

Most psychiatric conditions occur with similar frequency in all societies, but there are some syndromes unique to a single culture. They include:

1. Amok, in SE Asian men: an acute confusional state leading to murder and/or suicide.
2. Latah, in Malaysian women: a state of automatism precipitated by stress.

3. Koro, in young Chinese men: a state of panic caused by a delusion that the penis is disappearing.
4. Windigo psychosis, in N. American Indians: the patient believes he has turned into a monster, and cannibalizes other tribe members.

Immigration

Immigrants have a high psychiatric morbidity and are especially prone to develop paranoid states. Possible reasons for this are that pre-existing psychiatric abnormality could cause people to emigrate, that stressful life events such as political upheaval may force them to emigrate, and that arrival in the new country may cause 'culture shock', comprising strange language and customs, and discrimination against immigrants.

ORGANIZATION OF PSYCHIATRIC SERVICES

DHSS policy (Department of Health and Social Security, 1975) is to phase out mental hospitals, and introduce community care for the majority of psychiatric patients, with district general hospital (DGH) units for the minority who need inpatient treatment. Both community and inpatient treatment should be carried out by the multidisciplinary team approach.

This policy was introduced in the 1960s, but has only been partly implemented because of the high cost of transition from the old system.

The principle is that the mentally ill should be treated at home because this would be as effective as hospital care, and preferred by both patients and their families. The stigma of mental illness and the risk of institutionalization associated with the traditional mental hospital would be avoided, although the burden on patients' families probably increased.

DGH Units

DGH psychiatric units are part of the general hospital, sharing the same catchment area, usually 150,000–200,000 people.

Inpatient, day patient and outpatient facilities are provided. The unit is a base for staffing the community services. There is close collaboration between different departments, and patients can easily be transferred from one type of care to another.

Inpatient facilities comprise acute admission wards (30 beds per 60,000 population), medium stay wards, and rehabilitation wards.

The day hospital provides all the facilities available to inpatients during the day: medical and nursing care, occupational therapy, and access to specialized treatments like individual or group psychotherapy, behaviour therapy, and ECT. Inpatient and day patients may share the same facilities. The day hospital should be able to deal with most acute patients, except those for whom inpatient care is essential because of severe illness or unsuitable accommodation.

The outpatient department, as well as having general clinics, may provide clinics to monitor those on lithium or depot neuroleptics, and an emergency referral service.

Psychogeriatric patients should be provided with similar facilities, also sited in a DGH unit, but run separately.

DGH units make a consultation service with medicine, surgery, and obstetrics possible.

Criticisms of the DGH units are that their service is inappropriately modelled on medical ward practice; and that they are unsuitable for violent or persistently disturbed patients. The accumulation of patients who cannot live unsupported is causing blocked beds.

Other Recommended Treatment Services

1. Regional units for forensic psychiatry, adolescent psychiatry, alcoholism, and drug abuse.
2. Long-stay beds for demented patients.
3. Local authority hostels and day centres for chronic patients who do not need inpatient or daypatient care.

The problems of providing adequate psychiatric services are discussed by Clare (1980).

The Multidisciplinary Team

A 'multidisciplinary team' consists of one or more members of each professional group involved in psychiatric care: doctors, nurses, psychologists, social workers, and occupational therapists.

Each team member is involved in assessment and management of inpatients and day patients, each contributing both from a professional viewpoint and from personal knowledge of the patient.

It may be appropriate for one member of the team to treat a patient, but other members maintain some contact. Ultimate responsibility for patient care remains with the consultant in charge.

References

Clare, A. (1980). The contemporary state of psychiatry. In *Psychiatry in Dissent*. Tavistock, London.

Cooper, B., and Morgan, H. G. (1973). *Epidemiological Psychiatry*. Charles Thomas, Springfield, Illinois.

Cox, J. L. (1977). Review article: aspects of transcultural psychiatry. *Br. J. Psychiatry*, **130**, 211–221.

Department of Health and Social Security (1975). *Better Services for the Mentally Ill*. HMSO, London.

Editorial (1978). Life event stress and psychiatric illness. *Psychol. Med.*, **8**, 545–549.

Goldberg, D. P. (1972). *The Detection of Psychiatric Illness by Questionnaire*. Oxford University Press, London.

Hare, E. H., and Wing, J. K. (1970). *Psychiatric Epidemiology*. Oxford University Press, London.

Shepherd, M., Cooper, B., Brown, A. C., and Kalton, G. W. (1966). *Psychiatric Illness in General Practice*. Oxford University Press, London.

CHAPTER 24

The Mental Health Act

Parts IV and V of the Mental Health (England and Wales) Act of 1959 govern the compulsory admission, detention, and treatment of psychiatric patients, and are used when mental disorder causes serious risk to the health or safety of the patient or of others, and the patient refuses hospitalization.

Mental illness and severe subnormality may be dealt with under any Section of the Act in patients of any age. Mild subnormality and psychopathy can be dealt with under Section 60 or 65 in patients of any age; under the other Sections, patients with these conditions may only be admitted to hospital if they are under 21, and only detained until the age of 25.

About 10% of new admissions and 5% of all inpatients are detained under the Act.

Section 29 permits compulsory admission for observation for up to 72 hours. Two applications are required, one from any registered medical practitioner, the other from an approved social worker (Mental Welfare Officer) or from a relative of the patient. Both applicants must have seen the patient in the three days before admission. Section 29 should only be used in an emergency. It can be converted into a Section 25 or 26 by a recommendation from a doctor recognized by the local health authority as having special experience in the diagnosis or treatment of mental disorder (under Section 28 of the Act).

Section 25 permits compulsory admission for observation for up to 28 days. Three applications are required, one from a doctor who has known the patient previously and is usually the GP, one from a doctor recognized under Section 28, and one from an approved social worker or the patient's nearest relative. The applicants must have seen the patient in the 14 days before admission. The patient can only be discharged from the Section by the consultant psychiatrist responsible.

Section 26 permits detention for treatment for up to one year. It may be renewed for another year, and subsequently for two years at a time. The mental disorder must be one likely to respond to treatment. Three applications are required as for Section 25. The patient's nearest relative can arrange discharge from Section 26 by written notice to the hospital authorities, but the consultant responsible can overrule the relative's application. Either the patient or the nearest relative can appeal against the Section to a Mental Health Review Tribunal, consisting of a lawyer, a doctor, and a lay member from outside the hospital.

Section 30 permits an informal patient already in hospital to be detained for observation for up to 72 hours on the recommendation of one doctor, preferably the consultant responsible.

Section 60 permits a Court of Assize, Quarter Sessions, or Magistrates' Court to order the detention of a patient found guilty of a criminal offence in a specified hospital for up to a year, if supported by medical recommendations as for Section 25. The hospital must take the patient within 28 days. If the patient absconds for long enough (one month in the case of mental illness, six months in the case of psychopathy or subnormality) the Section lapses.

Section 65 can only be applied by a judge in a Court of Assize or Quarter Sessions. It is a hospital order for unlimited time which prevents discharge, transfer, or leave without the consent of the Home Secretary. The patient or the nearest relative may appeal to the Home Secretary against the Section but does not have access to a Mental Health Review Tribunal.

Section 135 permits a Mental Welfare Officer to obtain a warrant authorizing the police to remove a mentally disturbed person from any premises to a place of safety, usually a mental hospital, for observation for up to 72 hours.

Section 136 permits a police officer to take a person who appears to be suffering from a mental disorder to a place of safety, usually a mental hospital, for observation for up to 72 hours.

The Mental Health (Scotland) Act, 1960, employs similar principles but the Sections have different numbers; Section 31 governs emergency admissions for up to seven days on one medical recommendation,

Section 24 governs admission for longer periods on two medical recommendations.

Changes to the Mental Health Act

Compulsory treatment of the mentally ill is a source of controversy (Clare, 1980). Extreme critics think it should be abolished because psychiatric patients have a right to decide for themselves whether they want treatment. The opposite view is that it is in patients' best interests to be treated against their will when they are too disturbed to realize that treatment is necessary, especially if they are suicidal, or violent towards others, as a result of mental illness.

The white paper *A Review of the Mental Health Act 1959* (Department of Health and Social Security, 1978) recommends some changes to the present legislation. These include:

1. Treatment given without patients' consent should be more strictly controlled, especially if it is of 'irreversible, hazardous or not fully established' type.
2. Patients should have more information about their legal rights, and more opportunity to appeal about compulsory hospitalization and treatment.

Further Reading

A booklet produced by Wyeth (1980) summarizes the Mental Health Act, and operation of the Act is reviewed by Chiswick (1979).

References

Clare, A. (1980). Responsibility and compulsory hospitalisation. In *'Psychiatry in Dissent'*. Tavistock, London.

Chiswick, D. (1979). Operating the Mental Health Acts. *Br. J. Hosp. Med.* **21**, 167–175.

Department of Health and Social Security (1978). *A Review of the Mental Health Act 1959*. Cmnd. 7320. HMSO, London.

Wyeth Laboratories (1980). *A Glossary of Mental Disorders and Mental Health Legislation*. Wyeth, Maidenhead.

APPENDIX I

Case Histories

These case histories are intended to illustrate the presentation and course of some common psychiatric conditions for readers with limited clinical experience.

Schizophrenia

A 20 year old single girl in her second term at teacher training college was noted to be isolated from other students and was falling behind with her work. She told her tutor people were talking about her because her body was changing. During an interview with a student counsellor she talked vaguely and sometimes laughed for no apparent reason. Over the next few weeks she spent increasingly long periods in her room. Her GP was asked to visit; she did not reply to his questions, and sat smiling until he got up to leave, then knelt at his feet, cried 'Behold the Lamb of God' and wept uncontrollably. She was admitted to a psychiatric hospital, where she said she heard the voices of St. Anne and the Virgin Mary telling each other she was pregnant by the Lamb of God, and could feel her womb being divided into three by the Holy Trinity. Sometimes she appeared elated, wandering round the ward making the sign of the cross; at other times she sat on her bed giggling or weeping quietly.

Chlorpromazine (Largactil) 50 mg four times a day was given, and increased to 100 mg four times a day a week later. There was a gradual improvement over the next month in that she stopped talking about her hallucinations, could converse logically on other topics, and no longer required supervision to wash, dress, or eat; however, she said she still heard voices when questioned about them, and showed no initiative to do anything. She was transferred to a rehabilitation ward, and medication changed to flupenthixol decanoate (Depixol) 40 mg fortnightly. Six months later she left hospital to live in lodgings, and with encouragement to get up in the mornings was able to hold a job in a factory. Depixol injections were continued by the community nurse.

Paraphrenia

A 64 year old single retired canteen supervisor, who lived alone, was seen on a domiciliary visit. She believed that her neighbours were changing the taste of her food by directing electric currents through the walls, and heard them talking about her at night; she had complained to the police about them several times. Eventually she consulted her GP because the problems were 'upsetting her nerves'.

She was aggressive in manner, talked loudly and copiously, and although she did not look depressed reported depressive symptoms of interrupted sleep, poor appetite, and reduced concentration. Thought content was concerned with her neighbours' persecution, and paranoid delusions and auditory hallucinations as described above were present. Cognitive functions were intact.

The suggestion of hospital admission was indignantly refused, but she agreed to have a sleeping tablet and was prescribed trifluoperazine (Stelazine) 10 mg nightly. A month later she reported that the neighbours were now leaving her alone; after a further month, she described her former beliefs about them as just imagination. Follow-up was discontinued and she was advised to take the medication indefinitely.

Six months later, she was admitted to hospital after a large overdose of trifluoperazine, which she had stopped taking regularly. Her delusions and hallucinations had returned, and distressed her so much that she decided she would be better dead. After resuscitation she was transferred to the psychiatric ward, and started on fortnightly injections of fluphenazine decanoate (Modecate), 50 mg, which could be continued by the community nurse following her discharge.

Depressive Psychosis

A 66 year old retired headmaster was transferred to the psychiatric ward after treatment for a large overdose of amitriptyline. He had left a suicide note in which he apologized for causing the country so many problems, and asked his family to forgive him. He was discovered unconscious in a wood near his home. Intensive care was necessary because of cardiac arrhythmias but a week later he was physically recovered. He said he took the overdose because of guilt over having completed a tax return incorrectly ten years ago; he believed himself thereby responsible for the economic difficulties in Britain. For six months he had been waking at 3 a.m. each morning, had had very little appetite, lost weight and been very constipated, symptoms which he suspected were due to bowel cancer. He had lost interest in his former hobbies of reading and birdwatching. His GP had diagnosed a depressive illness and prescribed amitriptyline (Lentizol) 50 mg at night, increasing to 100 mg when there had been no response after a month, but he had still not improved two months later.

On examination he was thin and agitated, wringing his hands and fidgeting, unable to concentrate long enough to answer the interviewer's questions but continually apologizing for this. He was preoccupied with guilt over the tax return and the overdose. Cognitive testing was abandoned when he became distressed about what would happen if he gave the wrong answers.

ECT was thought necessary despite some concern about his fitness for anaesthetic. At first he refused it because 'it would be a form of torture' but eventually consented. After four treatments he was improving, and received eight in all; after the last two he became slightly confused, but this cleared in a few days. He remained well, enjoying his retirement, until his wife died the following year and then his depressive symptoms returned and only partly resolved with further ECT.

Manic-depressive Psychosis

A 30 year old single physiotherapist was admitted under Section 25 of the Mental Health Act. For three weeks she had, according to the friend with whom she shared a flat, been very active, rude, and irritable. She had sent several Valentine cards to a surgeon at the hospital where she worked, and that afternoon she had bought two air tickets to Paris, and told her friend she was going to elope with him. When the friend tried to stop her, she threw a knife in her face. The police who were called recognized the likelihood of mental illness and the GP, duty psychiatrist, and duty social worker who were asked to see her agreed that hospital admission was required.

She was very angry on arrival in the ward and threatened to sue the police force and medical profession for infringement of human rights. She tried to leave the ward as she said she was commissioned by Mrs. Thatcher to fly to Paris that night to do vital medical research.

Five years before she had had a manic illness followed by a severe episode of depression requiring ECT. She had subsequently had lithium carbonate to prevent further episodes, but stopped it two years later as she was gaining a lot of weight. Her mother had also had manic-depressive psychosis and had died by suicide when the patient was a baby.

Treatment with haloperidol, 10 mg four times a day, with the addition of procyclidine 5 mg as required to counteract Parkinsonian side-effects, made her much calmer after a few days but there were still aggressive outbursts, and she started to express fears that she was going to die from cancer soon. The possibility that she was swinging from the manic to the depressed phase led to the reduction of haloperidol to 5 mg twice daily, and lithium carbonate was prescribed in the form of Priadel 1000 mg daily. Her mood stabilized over the next fortnight but when she started to make plans for discharge she found she had lost her flat as a result of her behaviour, and realization of her conduct towards the surgeon made her decide to look for another job elsewhere. She was discharged to a hostel, still taking lithium and intending to continue it.

Depressive Neurosis

A 35 year old divorced nursing assistant was admitted after expressing suicidal thoughts to her GP. She had six months' history of depressed mood, difficulty getting off to sleep, diminished appetite, and frequent headaches, and attributed it all to living alone in a damp flat with noisy neighbours. The symptoms were worst when she was at home in the evenings, but were lessened by alcohol and she was drinking half a bottle of sherry each night. Her GP had prescribed diazepam (Valium), mianserin (Norval), and phenelzine (Nardil) in turn, but they all produced side-effects and none of them helped.

On admission she was drably dressed, subdued, and tearful, but gave a rational account of her problems. A week later, without medication, she was much improved. She took an active part in a ward discussion group, and said she had come to realize that drink would not solve her problems but she must make a positive effort to overcome them. Advised by the social worker, she applied to the council for rehousing, and was told that she would be allocated a better flat within a few months. Following discharge there was some recurrence of her depression and occasional excess drinking until she obtained her new flat, when she became much happier and remained so six months later.

Anxiety/Depressive Neurosis

A 24 year old housewife was referred to outpatients with six months' history of being afraid to go out shopping or on buses without her husband, feeling 'strung up' all the time, crying over little things, interrupted sleep, a lump in her throat which caused difficulty in swallowing, and loss of interest in sex. She had been married four years, described her husband as 'very understanding', and said there were no problems with him or their 3 year old daughter. Her own childhood had been unhappy as her parents were always quarrelling. A year before her father had died of heart disease, and since his death her mother had appeared hostile towards her.

Isocarboxazid (Marplan) 10 mg three times a day and diazepam (Valium) 10 mg at night were prescribed, and she agreed to attend outpatients fortnightly over the next few months. She was advised to go out alone for increasing distances each day and at each outpatient visit she brought a written record of her progress in doing so. She was also given the opportunity to express her grief about her father's death, and discuss ways in which she might improve her relationship with her mother. All her symptoms improved over the next six months and she was then gradually able to stop her medication and outpatient visits despite some reluctance to do so.

Obsessive–Compulsive Neurosis

A 28 year old housewife had four years' history of obsessive-compulsive symptoms. She had always been an anxious and methodical person, and after the birth of her only child was extremely particular about sterilizing his feeds correctly. When he had a minor gastro-intestinal upset one day, she became constantly troubled by the fear that he would die from food poisoning unless she kept all germs away from him, and evolved complex rituals for preparing his food, bathing him, and washing his clothes. She was aware that these rituals were unnecessary but could not stop herself carrying them out, and if her husband tried to stop her she reacted with outbursts of rage. Initially she had been treated with clomipramine, 200 mg daily for three months, then with phenelzine, 90 mg daily for three months, neither of which made any difference. An intensive programme of behaviour therapy, in which a psychologist spent long periods at home with her discouraging the rituals and encouraging other activities, helped only while the psychologist was present. A two year course of dynamic psychotherapy did not help either, and towards the end of it she became very depressed, and preoccupied with guilt about the effect of her symptoms on her family. By this time her husband, previously tolerant and supportive, was considering a separation so that he could apply for custody of their son. Her depressive symptoms lessened after 10 ECT, but the obsessive-compulsive symptoms were still unchanged.

She was referred to a centre which specialized in psychosurgery, and following a period of inpatient assessment there, underwent a leucotomy. This was followed by immediate relief of her symptoms. Two years later she was well and able to look after her home and family.

Personality Disorder, Antisocial Type

A 24 year old single man was admitted to the psychiatric ward from Casualty, having inflicted superficial cuts on both wrists after the girl with whom he lived had asked him to leave. He complained of constant tension sometimes leading to outbursts of anger he could not control, insomnia, headaches, and depressed mood.

His old notes showed that he had been born following a difficult breech delivery, and a slight weakness of the right leg had been present from birth. At school he performed badly although his IQ was found to be average, and he was often in trouble for stealing and lying. When he was 12 his father died in an accident and he subsequently became even more badly behaved. He attended a Child Guidance Clinic for some months but did not improve. Since leaving school at 16 he had had over 100 jobs, most of which had ended because of fights or arguments with workmates. He had had several girlfriends but several of these relationships had ended because he was violent towards them while drunk. He had previously been seen by a psychiatrist for a Court Report when charged with damage to an ex-girlfriend's house.

On admission he was tearful and judged to be moderately depressed, but became more cheerful in a few days, made friends with other patients, and was helpful to the ward staff. In view of his headaches and aggressive outbursts, he had a full neurological examination which showed only the old UMN lesion of his leg, and an EEG which showed bilateral slight temporal abnormalities of doubtful significance. Discharge from hospital was suggested to him but he said he had nowhere to go, became verbally aggressive and smashed a window. The duty doctor gave him 10 mg of diazepam (Valium) i.v. and he continued to demand this drug several times a day. When it was refused he suddenly discharged himself and was later found to be at another ex-girlfriend's home.

Alcoholism

A 38 year old unemployed man was referred by his GP to an alcoholism treatment unit. He had been drinking at least five pints of beer and five large whiskies daily for years, having started to drink regularly in the Royal Navy as a young man. Alcohol had helped him to forget the stresses of his job, and to mix better in social gatherings, and he was not aware that he might be drinking to excess. He left the Navy rather than apply for promotion, which he found a worrying prospect, and went into hotel management, continuing heavy regular social drinking in his new job. He would start the day with a glass of whisky, as without one he felt anxious and his hands tended to shake. His wife became concerned about the money spent on drink but he would not discuss this with her. He continued drinking after he was involved in a car accident with 120 mg/100 ml of alcohol in his blood and lost his licence. At age 34, he underwent emergency surgery for a perforated peptic ulcer and two days postoperatively became tremulous, confused, and suspicious, said he saw green frogs on his bed, and had a grand mal fit. Delirium tremens was diagnosed and treated with chlormethiazole (Heminevrin) 1000 mg thrice daily, phenobarbitone 30 mg thrice daily, and vitamin injections. Before leaving hospital he was told that he was an alcoholic and should stop drinking completely, and was given the addresses of the local branch of Alcoholics Anonymous and the Council on Alcoholism. He attended these organizations' meetings occasionally, but still drank heavily, attempts at abstinence resulting in tremulousness and anxiety which led him to take another drink after a few days. Eventually he was dismissed from his job, and his wife announced her intention to leave him. These two events changed his attitude, and he asked his GP to refer him to a specialized unit as he was determined to stop drinking and knew he needed help.

APPENDIX II

Glossary of Terms

Abreaction
The recall to consciousness of a repressed trauma, with a re-experiencing of the emotion which originally accompanied it. Methods of achieving abreaction ('catharsis') include psychotherapy alone, or psychotherapy aided by hypnosis or by drugs, usually barbiturates or amphetamines.

Acting out
Repetition of behaviour appropriate to an earlier stage of development, during psychotherapy.

Agitation
Motor restlessness, usually accompanied by subjective anxiety. Occurs in anxiety states and depressive illness.

Akathisia
Motor restlessness due to malfunction of the extrapyramidal system. A side-effect of neuroleptics.

Asyndetic thinking
There is no logical connection between one thought and the next. May occur in schizophrenia. (Synonymous with 'knight's move thinking'.)

Autism
(1) Autistic thinking: the subject is absorbed in personal fantasies or delusions, and thoughts are divorced from external reality. May occur in schizophrenia.
(2) Childhood autism: a form of childhood psychosis.

Autochthonous idea
An idea, usually delusional, which suddenly

182

enters consciousness fully formed for no apparent reason. Autochthonous delusions (synonymous with 'primary delusions') are first rank symptoms of schizophrenia.

Catatonia Mutism and immobility without impairment of consciousness. Occurs in schizophrenia.

Catharsis Achievement of abreaction.

Circumstantiality Excessively detailed and lengthy thought or talk which wanders around the point. Occurs in some epileptics and people of low intelligence.

Compulsion An obsessional act, which the subject carries out despite trying to resist doing so.

Confabulation Elaborate falsifications, probably believed by the subject, which cover up defects of memory. Occurs in amnesic states especially Korsakov's syndrome.

Conversion The manifestation of repressed emotion in the form of bodily symptoms. Occurs in hysteria.

Delusion An incorrigible false belief, inconsistent with the information available and with the beliefs of the subject's social group. Delusions may occur in the functional psychoses, and some organic states. Primary (autochthonous) delusions suddenly enter consciousness fully formed. They are sometimes preceded by a period of 'delusional mood'. They are a first rank symptom of schizophrenia. They may take the form of a delusional perception, developing in conjunction with an ordinary sense perception; a delusional memory; or a delusional awareness. Secondary delusions are often elaborated from them.
Paranoid delusions are the most common type.

Delusions in accord with the prevailing affect may occur in the affective disorders, e.g. delusions of guilt, nihilistic, or hypochondriacal delusions in depression, and grandiose delusions in mania. Other types are religious and sexual delusions.

Denial

An inability to accept a piece of self-knowledge, or an external event, of an unpleasant kind.

Depersonalization

A sensation of dreamlike unreality of the self. Usually secondary to an anxiety state or depressive illness, but may occur alone as the 'primary depersonalization syndrome' in young people.

Depression

(1) A mood state characterized by sadness, not necessarily pathological.
(2) Depressive illness.

Derealization

A sensation of dreamlike unreality of the outside world. Occurs in association with depersonalization.

Displacement

The transfer of emotion from the person or object which caused it towards a different but more acceptable one.

Dissociation

A splitting of consciousness in which one part of mental functioning becomes disconnected from the rest, e.g. a hysterical trance.

Echolalia and Echopraxia

The subject imitates the speech and actions of others.

Elation

Elevation of mood, including that seen in normal people, and that seen in mania or schizophrenia.

Euphoria

An exaggerated sense of well-being, usually indicating organic cerebral dysfunction.

Fixation

Arrest of one or more aspects of personality development at a stage of incomplete maturity.

Flight of ideas
Sudden changes in train of thought arising from incidental connections between words or ideas, like rhymes or puns. Occurs in mania.

Fugue
A state of altered consciousness in which the subject wanders away. May occur in depressive illness, hysteria, post-epileptic states, and after head injury.

Hallucination
A false perception arising in the absence of an appropriate external stimulus.
Hallucinations may occur in the functional psychoses, and some organic states.
They may involve any sensory modality: auditory, visual, tactile, somatic, olfactory, or gustatory types occur. Auditory ones in the form of voices are most frequent. Specific types of third person voices are first rank symptoms of schizophrenia. Second person voices are non-specific, but in the affective disorders the content tends to accord with the patient's mood.
Pseudohallucinations only occur in the visual and auditory modalities; they appear to be located in the subject's 'inner space' rather than to be coming from the external world; and the subject realizes they are not genuine perceptions.

Ideas of reference
Misinterpretation of external events as referring to the subject, usually in a derogatory way. Occur in paranoid states, but also in self-conscious young people without psychiatric illness.

Identification
Conscious or unconscious assumption of the characteristics of another person, usually someone admired by the subject.

Illusion
A perceptual distortion whereby a stimulus is misinterpreted. May occur in normal people or be secondary to mental illness.

Incongruity of affect	The subject's emotions are inappropriate to the circumstances. May occur in schizophrenia.
Introjection	Directing unpleasant emotions towards the self although they originated towards others.
Knight's move thinking	See asyndetic thinking.
Mannerisms	Artificial or exaggerated modes of speech or movement.
Negativism	Carrying out actions of an opposite nature to those requested.
Neologism	An idiosyncratic word which has a personal meaning for the subject but none for others. May occur in schizophrenia.
Neuroses	A group of psychiatric illnesses in which the symptoms may be viewed as representing an exaggeration of normal response to stress. Insight and contact with reality are usually retained. (Synonymous with 'psychoneuroses'.)
Obsession	A recurrent idea or impulse which enters consciousness despite resistance by the subject.
Overinclusive thinking	The subject's sense of concept boundaries is blurred so that ideas with little relevance to the topic are included, and thought becomes vague. May occur in schizophrenia.
Overvalued idea	An idea held with great conviction, but differing from a delusion in that it is not necessarily false, and the subject is to some extent prepared to modify it in response to evidence against it.
Paranoid states	Conditions in which delusions are the most prominent feature.
Passivity feelings	The subject believes that his thoughts,

emotions, or bodily actions are controlled by an outside agency. They are first rank symptoms of schizophrenia.

Perseveration	Continued repetition of speech or activity. Occurs in organic states.
Phobia	An excessive fear of a particular object or situation.
Pressure of speech	Rapid speech secondary to rapid thought of excess content. Occurs in mania.
Primary delusion	See 'delusion'.
Projection	Displacement of personal shortcomings or lack of success on to other people or outside factors, an unconscious method of avoiding guilt feelings.
Pseudohallucination	See 'hallucination'.
Psychoses	A group of psychiatric conditions in which the symptoms, e.g. delusions and hallucinations, are qualitatively different from normal experiences; and there is often loss of insight, loss of contact with reality, and deterioration of the general personality. 'Organic' psychoses result from physical factors affecting the brain, whereas in 'functional' psychoses the cause is unknown.
Rationalization	The subject explains his actions by a logical or admirable motive when the true one is not so acceptable.
Reaction formation	An unacceptable feeling is repressed, and the subject gives expression to its opposite.
Regression	A reversion to thoughts, feelings, or behaviour appropriate to an earlier stage of maturation.
Repression	Unacceptable thoughts or impulses are excluded from conscious awareness.

Retardation
(1) Psychomotor retardation; slowing of speech and motor activity.
(2) Mental retardation: synonymous with mental handicap.

Stereotypy
A meaningless, bizarre action or statement repeated frequently. May occur in schizophrenia.

Sublimation
The redirection of frustrated desires into socially acceptable channels.

Thought block
A sensation of the train of thought being suddenly interrupted. Occurs in schizophrenia, but is difficult to distinguish from the impairment of thought processes which may result from poor concentration in other conditions.

Thought interference
The subject's thoughts appear to be inserted into or withdrawn from his mind, or broadcast outside it, by some external agency. It is a first rank symptom of schizophrenia.

Transference
Feelings which the subject experienced towards someone in the past are inappropriately projected on to another person. It is often used in the context of a patient's feelings towards a psychotherapist.

Verbigeration
Constant repetition of a single word or phrase. May occur in schizophrenia.

Word salad
A mixture of neologisms which renders speech quite incomprehensible. May occur in schizophrenia.

Index